LIPPINCOTT'S
NEED-TO-KNOW

Research
Survival Guide

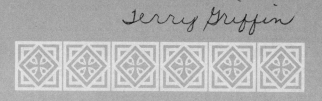

Terry Griffin

LIPPINCOTT'S
NEED-TO-KNOW

Research
Survival Guide

Ann Marttinen Doordan, PhD, RN
Professor
School of Nursing
San Jose State University
San Jose, California

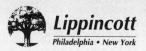

Lippincott
Philadelphia • New York

Acquisitions Editor: Margaret Zuccarini
Assistant Editor: Sara Lauber
Project Editor: Gretchen Metzger
Production Manager: Helen Ewan
Production Coordinator: Nannette Winski
Design Coordinator: Kathy Kelley–Luedtke
Indexer: Lynne Mahan

9 8 7 6 5 4 3 2 1

Library of Congress Cataloging-in-Publications Data

Doordan, Ann Marttinen.
    Lippincott's need-to-know : research survival guide / Ann Marttinen Doordan.
        p.   cm. — (Lippincott's need-to-know)
    ISBN 0-7817-1040-5 (alk. paper)
    1. Nursing—Research. 2. Nursing—Research—Terminology.
I. Title. II. Series.
    [DNLM: 1. Nursing Research—methods. 2. Research Design—nurses' instruction.   WY 20.5 D691L 1998]
RT81.5.D65   1998
610.73′072—dc21
DNLM/DLC
for Library of Congress   97-13229
                                               CIP

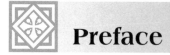

Preface

This book is designed to serve as a convenient reference to research and research terminology for both the novice and the more experienced researcher. The main feature is the comprehensive glossary of over 1000 terms used in research, theory, and statistics. The overview of research provides a framework for understanding the research process, obtaining on-line information, and developing a research report or proposal.

In Part One, the first section includes an overview of research, including a comparison of philosophic approaches to research. The section on preparation for research includes helpful guides to accessing and critiquing the research literature in print or electronic form. Selected internet addresses are given for on-line access to statistics, literature, and funding sources. The next sections compare quantitative and qualitative designs and analyses, including comprehensive classification and definition of research terminology, instrumentation, statistical techniques, and software packages. The section on dissemination of results provides guidelines for writing a research report, submission of a manuscript for publication or an abstract for presentation, and preparation of a research poster. The final section presents an overview for writing a research proposal, including a budget request.

Part Two is a comprehensive glossary of over 1000 research, theory, and statistical terms related to nursing research. The convenience of having the terminology all in one reference source appeals to beginning and advanced researchers, consumers of research, and students of research at the undergraduate and graduate level.

Part Three includes selected tables and examples for help with research consent, literature search, qualitative and quantitative research comparison, instrumentation, statistical symbols and information, and guidelines for critique of research studies.

I hope this reference will become a well-used and helpful addition to your library. It is intended to be a user-friendly portable resource for understanding and using nursing research.

Ann Marttinen Doordan, PhD, RN

Contents in Brief

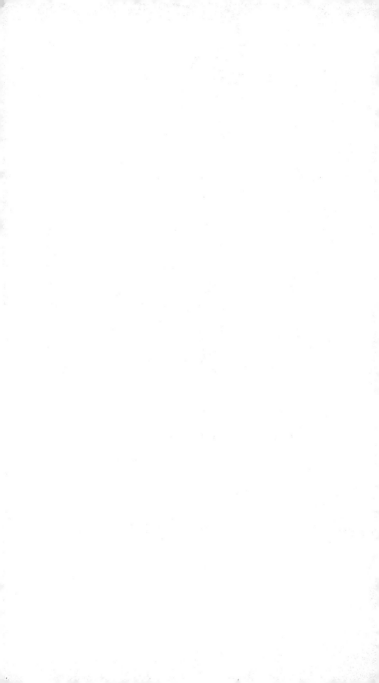

Contents

Index   181

*Unless otherwise noted, material in Part Three is
courtesy of:*

**Polit, D., Hungler, B. *Essentials of Nursing Research,
4/E.* Philadelphia: Lippincott, 1997.**

Sample Consent Form, p. 1135

Major Assumptions of the Positivist and Naturalistic Para-
digms, p. 13

Research Purposes and Research Questions, p. 19

Examples of Question Types, p. 258, Table 9–1

Guide to Widely Used Multivariate Statistical Analysis,
p. 360, Table 11–16

Outcomes of Statistical Decision Making, p. 340, Figure
11–7

**Polit, D., Hungler, B. *Nursing Research: Principles
and Methods, 5/E.* Philadelphia: Lippincott, 1997.**

Flow of Tasks in Analyzing Quantitative Data, p. 496,
Figure 21–1

Dimensions of Quantitative Research Designs, p. 155,
Table 6–1

Fictitious Example of a Cover Letter for a Mailed Questionnaire, p. 286, Figure 13–5

Examples of Concepts Frequently Measured With Composite Scales, p. 285, Table 13–4

Example of a Semantic Differential, p. 283, Figure 13–4

Example of a Likert Scale to Measure Attitudes Toward the
Mentally Ill, p. 282, Table 13–3

Example of a Checklist, p. 279, Figure 13–1

Summary of Statistical Tests, pp. 424–425, Table 18–6

Relationships of Central Tendency Indexes in Skewed Distributions, p. 382, Figure 17–5

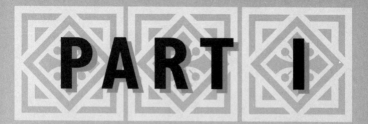

PART I

Elements
of Nursing
Research

Introduction to Nursing Research

Nursing has a long research history and tradition. Florence Nightingale systematically collected statistics on factors associated with disease and observed the positive effects of new hygienic and cleanliness procedures on healing. The focus shifted to nursing education research as the profession evaluated nursing education and professional roles. Since the 1950s, more clinical nursing research has been conducted. In 1993, the National Institute for Nursing Research was established in the National Institutes for Health to further the nursing research agenda. Nurses are consumers and producers of research that guides practice, education, and further research.

Philosophic Approaches to Research Methods

There are two philosophic approaches to nursing research, the empirical approach and the naturalistic approach. The *empirical* approach to science focuses on the collection and measurement of objective observations through one of the senses, such as vision or hearing. The *naturalistic* approach focuses on collection of information about the perspectives and meanings of experiences from the perspective of the individuals or groups directly living the experience. The empirical approach is *quantitative,* and numbers are used to test theory or specific theoretical relationships. The naturalistic approach uses *qualitative* methods to gather information in the natural setting to increase understanding about experience or to develop a theory about the topics of interest. Both approaches are needed in nursing.

Purpose of Nursing Research

The discipline of nursing involves complex relationships among the *client,* the *nurse, health,* and the *environment.*

Nursing research attempts to understand these complex human relationships to generate knowledge that will improve nursing practice, education, and research. Empirical and naturalistic approaches are used at each level to develop knowledge for understanding and controlling events.

BASIC AND APPLIED RESEARCH. The purpose of research is to develop knowledge (basic research) or to find solutions for problems (applied research). *Basic research* is conducted to develop theory and a knowledge base, which may or may not have immediate clinical application. *Applied research* is conducted to develop solutions for clinical problems, which in turn may suggest basic research questions.

Overview of Nursing Research

The research process is a systematic approach to gather information to *describe, explore, explain,* or *predict* phenomena of interest. *Phenomena* are topics that can be events, behaviors, happenings, or situations in nursing and health care. Phenomena that vary and can be measured are called *variables. Subjects* are the individuals or groups who serve as informants or participants in the research, and the *researcher* designs and conducts the study.

Concepts are terms used to describe abstract ideas and build theory. A *theory* is an abstract explanation of reality. Research is used to test theory through empirical quantitative methods or to develop theory through naturalistic qualitative methods.

Quantitative Research

Quantitative research is based on the empirical approach to research. It is the study of phenomena that can be objectively measured and quantified. Numbers and statistics are used to describe the frequency with which some attribute occurs or to explore whether two variables are related to one another. The attributes are measured with instruments that yield scores or values to describe the variance of the attribute, such as the frequency or quantity of the attribute. Quantitative studies are also used to explain how an attribute causes an outcome or how to predict (control) an outcome through an intervention. A *causal* variable is called an *independent variable* and the *effect* (outcome) is called a *dependent variable*. In an experiment, the researcher implements an intervention (the cause or independent variable) and studies how it affects the outcome (the effect or dependent variable). The data are statistically analyzed to describe the distribution, frequency, or magnitude and reliability of the relationships among phenomena. The research uses a controlled design following strict rules of scientific methodology.

PHASES OF A QUANTITATIVE STUDY. A quantitative study is composed of three phases: conceptualization and design; data collection and analysis; and discussion, conclusion, and reporting. In the first phase, the researcher identifies the research topic, purpose, and key concepts to be explored and defines the research problem. After a comprehensive review of the literature to explore the problem further, a conceptual or theoretical framework may be specified. Then a research question or hypothesis is formed to guide the research study. The design consists of the plan to answer the research question or test the hypothesis. It includes the plan of how to measure (operationalize) the concepts of interest, what type of research design is necessary to answer the question or test the hypothesis, who will participate and how they will be selected, what setting will be used, what data collection procedures will be used, and how the data will be analyzed. Permission to conduct the study is obtained from the setting, and the proposal is submitted to an institutional review board (IRB) for approval to conduct the study.

In the data collection and analysis phase, data are collected from subjects after they consent to participate in the study. Data are collected with valid and reliable instruments designed to measure the variables of interest. The data from the instruments are prepared for analysis through review for completion and for necessary coding. They are then entered into a computer to form a data base for analysis through statistical procedures. The statistical tests are conducted and the results reviewed for completion.

In the discussion, conclusion, and reporting phase, the statistical findings are interpreted and discussed in relation to the framework and conceptual foundation for the study. Conclusions are drawn to summarize the results of the study. The conclusion may include limitations of the study, implications for nursing practice, and recommendations for practice and research. The results are disseminated in written reports or oral presentations.

Qualitative Research

Qualitative research is the systematic study of phenomena as they naturally occur in the field setting without intervention by the researcher. Qualitative research is based on the naturalistic approaches to research. Qualitative methods are used to describe the meaning or importance of the phenomena or to explore the development of the phenomena. Information is obtained from people in the natural setting. Qualitative studies can also be used to explain further the meaning and development of the phenomena to build theory about them.

PHASES OF A QUALITATIVE STUDY. A qualitative study consists of three phases, similar to the phases of a quantitative study: conceptualization, data collection and analysis, and conclusion and reporting. In the conceptualization phase, the researcher identifies the phenomena to be observed and general questions to be answered. The researcher may choose to avoid a review of literature to remain free from the bias of other studies of the phenomena. Then a design for the study is developed with identification of participants, setting, data collection, role of the researcher, and a plan for analysis of the information obtained. Permission to conduct the study is obtained from the setting, and the research proposal is submitted to an IRB for approval to conduct the study.

In the data collection and analysis phase, the researcher conducts the research in the natural (field) setting. The researcher may be an active participant in a group or a nonparticipant observer and may or may not disclose the purpose of the study or the identity of the researcher, according to the purpose of the study. The data are collected and analyzed until further data collection reveals no new ideas or themes and the data have been saturated. The descriptive data are organized and synthesized with qualitative methods to allow patterns of relationships and the meaning of the data to emerge. These patterns are systematically summarized and interpreted by the researcher.

In the conclusion phase, the summarized results may be compared with the review of literature, the implications of the findings are discussed, and recommendations are made for practice and research. The results are disseminated in written manuscripts or oral presentations.

Preparation for Research

Prior to developing the design, the researcher refines the research questions and conducts an extensive review and critique of the literature. The ethical considerations are reviewed prior to selecting the design.

Research Problems, Questions, and Hypotheses

The *purpose* of the research is to describe a phenomenon or to answer a research question. Research questions and problems emerge from clinical practice, professional literature, social events, testing of theory, or experience. The researcher identifies a topic of interest and a general or specific research purpose. During this phase, the researcher determines whether the problem is significant, researchable, and feasible to study. The researcher may review the literature and discuss the problem with colleagues to refine further the *statement of the problem*.

The researcher identifies the *research question*, which may be written as a statement or a question. If the researcher is able to make a prediction about the relationship between variables, a *research hypothesis* is written to state the predicted relationship. It may state that there is a relationship or predict the direction of the relationship. For example, the hypothesis may state that an increase in one variable will correspond to an increase in the second variable.

Review of Literature

A comprehensive review of literature is conducted to identify and critique what is already known about the research topic, to determine what gaps or questions remain to be studied, and to clarify the research question. The review can begin with a computerized data base available on disk or through the internet or with written indexes to research literature. Types of research literature include reports of thesis or dissertation studies; final reports to funding agencies sponsoring research, books, or professional or special interest journals; and proceedings from research symposia. Some refereed journals focus primarily on publication of research reports, such as *Advances in Nursing Science, Image, Nursing Research, Research in Nursing and Health,* and *Rehabilitation Nursing Research.* Other journals publish other specialty literature and one or two research reports per issue, such as *Archives of Psychiatric Nursing, Heart and Lung, Journal of Advanced Nursing, Journal of Cardiovascular Nursing, Journal of Family Nursing, Journal of Nursing Education, Maternal-Child Nursing,* and multiple other specialty journals.

Some qualitative researchers prefer not to conduct an extensive review of the literature prior to the study to avoid possible bias or preconceived interpretations of the phenomena. In this situation, they may conduct the review of literature after data analysis is complete to compare and discuss their findings relative to what is already known about the topic.

COMPUTERIZED LITERATURE SEARCH. A computer search can be conducted with a CD-ROM, a disk containing the information, on-line to a computerized data base, or on-line through the internet. Librarians with expertise can help with the search, sometimes for a fee, or the researcher can conduct the search free or for a fee for certain databases. One of the most widely used databases for nursing literature, the Cumulative Index to Nursing and Allied Health Literature (CINAHL) is available in print, on CD-ROM, or through the internet.

COMMONLY USED INDEXES. Searches can be organized around a subject, related subjects, key words, or author's names and can be narrowed by language, year of publication, research only, or by other factors to provide a broad or narrow search. Commonly used indexes include the following:

CINAHL	Cumulative Index to Nursing and Allied Health Literature
ERIC	Educational Resources Information Center
Health	Health Planning and Administration
MEDLINE	Medical Literature On-Line
PsychLIT	Psychology Literature
SCISEARCH	Science Search
SOCIALSCISEARCH	Social Science Search

CRITIQUING INTERNET INFORMATION. A large amount of additional information is available on the internet. Because anyone can post information on the internet without peer review, the information must be carefully critiqued. Several questions should be asked: Is the information credible and logical? Is full citation given for the source of information? Is there any supporting evidence for claims? Are the credentials and reputation of the author given? Is the information current?

WORLD WIDE WEB SITES. Several web sites offer helpful statistical information, resource information for researchers, network opportunities among researchers, and information on research, funding, or education. Directories and search engines, such as AltaVista, Infoseek, MedWeb, or Yahoo!, help in locating web sites. It is not possible to obtain free access to complete journal articles due to copyright restrictions. The following sites, available free or with fees, are helpful to researchers:

http://www.ahcpr.gov/
  Agency for Health Care Policy and Research

http://www.cdc.gov/cdc.html
  Centers for Disease Control and Prevention

http://cinahl.com/
  CINAHL Information Systems

http://www.cc.emory.edu/WHSCL/medweb.html
  Emory University's MedWeb: Biomedical Internet Resources

http://www.os.dhhs.gov:80/progorg/grantsnet
/index.html
  Health and Human Services Grantline

http://igm.nlm.nih.gov
  Internet GratefulMed

http://www.mnrs.org
  Midwest Nursing Research Society

http://www.cdc.gov/nchswww/nchshome.htm
  National Center for Health Statistics

http://nhic-nt.health.org/
  National Health Information Center

http://www.nih.gov/
  National Institutes of Health

http://www.med.nyu.edu//nih-guide.html
  National Institutes of Health-Guide to Grants and
  Contracts Database

http://www.nih.gov/ninr/
  National Institute of Nursing Research

http://www.nnln.nlm.nih.gov/
  National Network of Libraries of Medicine

http://stti-web.iupui.edu/
  Sigma Theta Tau International Nursing Honor Society

Research Critique

A critique is a critical evaluation of the strengths and
weaknesses of a study. A critique is conducted prior to
use of results in practice or research and when conducting
a review of literature. The framework, operational definitions, measurements, methodology, analysis, limitations,
conclusions, and presentation of the study are examined
for logic, consistency, accuracy, adherence to rules guid-
ing analysis, objectivity, ethical considerations, validity, reliability, and generalizability of the results.

A refereed journal publishes articles that have been reviewed and critiqued by experts prior to acceptance for
publication. The qualifications of the researcher also are
important to check. In conducting a review of literature, it
is best to use primary reports of the study rather than another person's summary of the results. Some journals only
publish short summaries, or briefs, which do not provide
much information on the study design and procedures. An
article may consist of a summary of ideas or opinions
rather than a scholarly report of research.

Ethical Considerations

The conduct of human research, which has the potential
to infringe on human rights, has resulted in the development of ethical guidelines for research by several disciplines and agencies, nationally and internationally. In
1975, the American Nurses Association published the

Human Rights Guidelines for Nurses in Clinical and Other Research.

ETHICAL DILEMMAS. Any study involving humans has a potential to pose an ethical dilemma. For example, the research role may conflict with the nurse role, probing for sensitive information may be traumatic, or withholding treatment from a control group may increase risk. As a nurse functions in the research role to gather data, some of the information may call for a nursing intervention that could interfere with the research results.

ETHICAL GUIDELINES. Ethical guidelines are general statements related to beneficence, dignity, and justice. The principle of *beneficence* is to avoid harm, avoid exploiting subjects, and minimize risk and maximize benefit in the risk/benefit ratio. In preserving *dignity,* subjects receive full disclosure of the risks, benefits, and procedures of the study; voluntarily participate; and provide informed consent to participate. *Justice* entails the fair treatment of subjects, equal opportunity to participate, protection of privacy through coding of information, reporting of aggregate data, and assurance of anonymity. Vulnerable groups are those who have limited ability to provide informed consent or are at greater risk of harm and require special protection to ensure preservation of their rights. Some examples include children, developmentally disabled people, pregnant women, the institutionalized, and the mentally ill or impaired.

Institutional Review Board

All institutions receiving government funding for research have an IRB, sometimes called the Human Subjects Review Board. The composition of the panel varies, usually consisting of a cross-section of researchers, lay people, ethicists, health providers, or social scientists. The board is responsible for the review of research proposals to ensure that each of the human rights is preserved, including that risk is minimized and safety is maximized, the research is reasonable and equitable, subjects are informed and have consent, privacy and confidentiality are assured, and vulnerable subjects are protected. Most boards provide guidelines for the preparation of the proposal for review that focus primarily on potential risk and procedures to collect and report data.

Research Designs

The design for the research study depends on the purpose of the study, presence or absence of a treatment, measurement of the variables, sample accessibility, and availability of resources for the conduct and analysis of the study. The following sections present an overview of the types of quantitative and qualitative designs, measurement principles, and sample selection strategies.

Quantitative Research Designs

Quantitative research designs allow the researcher to measure phenomena with numbers. The designs may be experimental, quasi-experimental, or nonexperimental. In each of the designs, the researcher attempts to control for other factors that may influence the results (dependent variable) with sample selection procedures or with statistical analysis. Threats to the *internal validity* occur when other factors besides the independent variable have an effect on the dependent variable. Factors such as history, selection bias, maturation, or mortality of subjects can have an effect. *External validity* or generalizability of the results is affected when subjects change because they are in a research situation. Random sampling and comparison with control groups attempt to control for some of these effects.

CONTROL METHODS. *Control methods* are implemented to reduce the amount of variance caused by external or intrinsic factors. Controlling factors in the environment and time factors, ensuring clear communication, following research protocols, and training research assistants decrease external variance. Intrinsic variance is controlled through randomization, homogeneity of subjects in the sample through use of exclusion and inclusion criteria, use of a block design, matching of subjects in the experimental and comparison groups, and the statistical technique of analysis of covariance.

EXPERIMENTAL RESEARCH. In true experimental research, subjects are *randomly assigned* to treatment groups, there is a *treatment* (manipulation of an independent variable), and there is a *control* group for comparison. With randomization, each member of the population has an equal chance of being selected for the study and of being assigned to the treatment group or the experimental group. The types of studies include a pretest/post-test, after only, factorial, repeated measures, and clinical trials. To be experimental, each design must include randomization, control, and an experimental treatment.

In the pretest/post-test control design, a baseline measure is taken on both groups before the treatment and repeated after the treatment. In the after only, the comparison between groups is made after one group receives the treatment. In the factorial design, subjects are randomly assigned to a treatment combination. Each treatment is a factor that must have at least two levels. Therefore, two variables with three levels (intensity of treatment, for example) results in a 2×3 factorial experiment. A repeated measures design tests variation in the same person who receives random order treatments; the subject serves as his or her own control. A clinical trial is a pretest/post-test control group design used to test clinical treatments experimentally.

QUASI-EXPERIMENTAL RESEARCH. If it is not feasible or ethical to conduct an experimental design, a quasi-experimental design is used. In this design, there is an experimental treatment, but a nonequivalent control group or no randomization occurs. Quasi-experimental designs include a nonequivalent control group design, in which data are obtained from one group and a non-equivalent group before and after a treatment, and a time series design, in which data are obtained from one group at several points before and after the treatment. The results after treatment are compared with results before the treatment in the same group of subjects. Pre-experimental studies are sometimes classified as quasi-experimental studies. These include a one-group before and after design (no control group) and a nonequivalent control group after only design.

NONEXPERIMENTAL RESEARCH. Nonexperimental designs include descriptive, retrospective, prospective, correlational, and case control studies. A descriptive study identifies factors present at one point. Retrospective studies are ex post facto studies in which the researcher identifies a current phenomenon and collects data from the past in an attempt to identify possible causal factors. Prospective studies are a type of longitudinal study in which a group of subjects with a condition at the present time is followed over time to identify outcomes. Correlational studies are used to examine the relationship between two variables. A case control study is a descriptive study of a group of subjects with a condition compared to a group of subjects without the condition.

OTHER QUANTITATIVE DESIGNS. Cross-sectional studies are nonexperimental studies conducted at one point, such as a retrospective study or a study in which data are collected from different age or developmental groups to examine differences on a variable. A longitudinal study is a nonexperimental prospective study that follows a group for a long period or is conducted as a follow-up of an earlier study.

Other types of quantitative studies include surveys to collect self-report information, needs assessments prior to development of a policy or program, program evaluation research, and methodology studies to examine the validity and reliability of instruments. Meta-analyses are studies that use statistical procedures to examine the results of a group of studies on the same topic.

Qualitative Research Designs

Qualitative studies use narrative forms of data, usually collected in the natural setting. The stories that emerge from the subjects are analyzed for patterns and themes. Types of qualitative designs include grounded theory, ethnography, phenomenology, hermeneutics, historical inquiry, ethical inquiry, feminist inquiry, critical social inquiry, and case studies.

GROUNDED THEORY. In grounded theory, which originated in sociology, subjects are observed as they interact in the social setting. The researcher may or may not participate actively in the group, and the subjects may or may not be aware that a research study is being conducted. The researcher collects field notes to record observations for later analysis. Interviews may be conducted to gather information.

ETHNOGRAPHY. In ethnographic research, which originated in anthropology, the researcher observes the behaviors and conversations of cultural groups in the natural (field) setting. Information is obtained on the meanings and patterns of the participants' experiences. The researcher becomes immersed in the culture to gain an understanding of their view of the world.

PHENOMENOLOGY AND HERMENEUTICS. Phenomenology and hermeneutics come primarily from philosophy. The goal is to understand the meaning and interpretation of the perceptions of lived experiences. The researcher conducts in-depth discussions with people experiencing a phenomenon to understand what that experience means to the person.

HISTORICAL INQUIRY. Historical inquiry focuses on the documents, records, films, and oral or written reports from people living at a period of time to interpret a past event from the perspective of that time period. Ethical inquiry examines ethical dilemmas and situations to examine the application of ethical principles and theories. Feminist inquiry studies problems relevant to women and women's experiences. Critical social inquiry critically analyzes the status of phenomena and alternatives to increase autonomy and responsibility. A case study is an analysis of an individual, family, or other group in the natural setting.

Multimethod Research

Multimethod research is undertaken when a researcher wants to obtain objective information along with more depth. For example, narrative data on how people perceive an experience can be collected through an interview, along with collection of quantitative data measured with an instrument.

Sampling Designs

Selection of the sample includes the use of *probability samples* or *convenience samples*. Experimental studies require probability samples, which include simple random, proportionate, stratified, cluster, and systematic sampling. *Simple random sampling* occurs when subjects are randomly selected and assigned to groups. The sample can be selected in *proportions* similar to the population proportion or from *strata* (segments in the population) to ensure representation on some attribute. *Cluster sampling* is selection of samples from large, then progressively smaller, clusters in the population. *Systematic sampling* occurs when the sample is selected according to predetermined intervals, such as every fifth person. Each of these methods yields a probability sample that is representative of the population.

Convenience samples are frequently used in quasi-experimental and nonexperimental research. A convenience sample includes subjects most available and convenient to study. A descriptive or qualitative study might use *snowball* sampling, a method in which one participant provides the names of other people with the same attribute. *Quota sampling* increases representation by using quotas to determine the number of people needed for each group. Convenience sampling techniques are used to obtain the quotas. In *purposive sampling,* the researcher selects subjects to be included in the sample according to personal judgment or prior knowledge.

Sample Size

Power analyses are conducted to determine the size of a sample for an experimental or quasi-experimental study. They use statistical procedures that take into account the effect size of the treatment and the number of variables to be measured in determining the size of the sample.

Qualitative studies and descriptive studies may be designed to be limited to a certain number of subjects or cases. In qualitative studies, data are collected until no new themes occur. At that point, the data are saturated and considered complete.

Measurement and Analysis of Data

Once the data are collected, they are systematically analyzed with methods consistent with the type of data available and the design for the study.

Measurement

Measurement is the quantification of variance. As a phenomenon changes in frequency, magnitude, or other quality, the changes are measured in numbers. In measurement, the obtained score is a function of the true score plus/minus the error score. Error occurs due to instrumentation, administration techniques, subject bias, observer bias, or situational bias. To control some of the instrumentation error, written instruments are checked for validity and reliability. Mechanical error is controlled through regular calibration and cross-checking of instruments. Careful instructions to the subjects, training of the observer, and control of extraneous environmental distractions all reduce the error.

Instruments are evaluated for the degree of reliability and validity. *Reliability* is the degree of consistency in measurement, such as calibrating a tool to ensure consistency. *Stability* is examined through test–retest reliability. *Internal consistency* (homogeneity) is assessed with Cronbach's alpha coefficient, in which each item is simultaneously compared with the other items in an instrument; item to total correlation; Kuder-Richardson *(KR-20)* coefficient estimate of homogeneity with dichotomous response instruments; or with split-half reliability, in which each half of an instrument is compared with the other half of the items. *Equivalence* is determined if the instrument yields similar results as another measure of the same construct on the same subjects. *Inter-rater* reliability is established by comparing the scores of two independent raters scoring the same phenomenon with the same subject.

Validity is the degree that an instrument measures what it is supposed to measure. The weakest form of validity is *face* validity, a judgment that the instrument looks like it measures what it intends to measure. *Content* validity is that the instrument adequately samples all aspects of the phenomenon it is intended to measure. *Criterion*-related validity is a comparison of the scores with external criteria resulting in a validity coefficient. *Concurrent* validity is the ability of the instrument to measure differences among individuals with different values of the phenomenon. *Predictive* validity is the ability of the instrument to predict accurately a future outcome. *Construct* validity is an assessment of what the instrument is measuring. It is obtained through factor analysis to identify the clusters within the instrument or with testing on known groups, in which the test is given to subjects with known differences in the attribute. *Convergent* validity indicates agreement between the scores obtained with two measures of the same construct given to the same group of subjects. *Divergent* validity is obtained through comparison with results obtained with an instrument that measures the opposite of the construct.

Qualitative Evaluation

The observations in qualitative research are evaluated for *credibility* and trustworthiness through methods such as prolonged engagement, persistent observation, triangulation of data sources or methods, member checks, peer debriefings, negative case analysis, and researcher credibility. *Dependability* is a check of stability through analysis by separate groups or an external audit. *Confirmability* is the agreement through an audit by an independent investigator. *Transferability* is the ability of the results to apply to another situation.

Sources of Data

Data can be collected from existing records, or new data can be generated. *Existing records* include charts, historical records, or data from a prior study. New data can be obtained through self-report measures, biotechnology, or observations. *Self-report* measures include interview guides, life histories, group discussions, critical incident recall, written diaries, questionnaires, semantic differential or analog scales, or Q-sort techniques. *Biotechnology* is used to obtain measurements of the body (in vivo) through spirometers, thermometers, electrocardiogram machines, or other instrumentation, or to measure samples outside the body (in vitro) through blood, body fluid, or other analysis. *Observations* are recorded verbally or in writing, sometimes on instruments or scales that measure the phenomena. Observers may intervene or observe without intervention and may be concealed or open about the research role.

Quantitative Analysis

Quantitative measurement is classified into four levels: nominal, ordinal, interval, and ratio. *Nominal* measurement, the lowest level, consists of assignment into categories. Numbers may be used as arbitrary codes for the categories, such as 1 for men and 2 for women. With *ordinal* level measurement, scores or objects are ranked in relative order, and the intervals between ranks are not specified. Class rank is an ordinal measure. *Interval* measurement is obtained with rank order and specified distance between rank, with an arbitrary 0, such as Fahrenheit temperature. The intervals between each level are equal. *Ratio* measurement, the highest level, consists of rank order, equal interval data based on an absolute zero. An example of a ratio measure is weight. The level of measurement determines the type of statistical procedures, with more analytic possibilities for interval and ratio data than for nominal or ordinal data. It is more powerful, for example, to work with an exact weight than with categories of weight above or below a certain number.

The two types of statistics are descriptive and inferential statistics. *Descriptive statistics* can be univariate (one variable) or bivariate (two variables). Univariate statistics include *frequency distributions,* measures of *central tendency* (mean, median, and mode), and *standard deviation* or range of measures to describe the degree of variation. Bivariate statistics include *contingency tables* and *correlations.* Product moment correlations are used with data at the interval and ratio level of measurement, and Spearman's rank order correlations are used with ordinal level data.

Inferential statistics are based on laws of probability. The researcher draws inferences about the population based on information obtained with a sample. Statistics allow the researcher to examine the variance in the sample to determine whether the amount of sampling error allows reliable estimates. Inferential statistics are based on sampling distributions. The *sampling distribution of the mean* is a theoretical distribution of samples from the same population. The *standard error of the mean* is the standard deviation (variance) of the theoretical distribution. A sample with a small standard deviation provides more reliable estimates of the population values.

Statistical procedures test the *null hypothesis,* which means that any observed difference is due to chance. Acceptance of the null hypothesis means that there is no difference, and rejection means that there is a difference between the variables measured. A *type I* error is incorrect rejection of the null hypothesis, or rejection when the null hypothesis is true: There is no difference. A *type II* error is acceptance of the null hypothesis when it should be rejected, because there is a difference. The level of significance, the alpha level, is the probability of committing a type I error. A .05 level of significance is the chance that only 5 out of 100 samples would reject the null hypothesis when it should have been accepted. Statistical significance means that the results are due to a difference at the probability level of .05.

Parametric statistical tests are based on the assumption of a normal distribution and the use of interval or ratio level measurement. The *t-test,* which measures differences between groups, and *analysis of variance,* which measures differences within and between groups, are the most commonly used parametric tests.

Nonparametric statistical tests, which are less powerful than parametric tests, use nominal or ordinal data and do not require normal distributions. *Chi-square* tests, which measure differences in categories and proportions, and *Pearson's r,* which measures differences in correlations, are commonly used nonparametric tests.

Multivariate statistics test the relationship among three or more variables. *Multiple regression* tests relationships among two or more independent variables on a dependent variable. The multiple correlation coefficient estimates the proportion of variance in the dependent variable explained by the independent variable. *Factor analysis* is a method to identify common factors among a set of variables. *Path analysis* is used to test the strength of relationships and order of relationships among multiple factors.

Qualitative Analysis

Qualitative analysis is systematic and organized but does not have the same set of firm rules that govern quantitative analyses. The type of analysis varies with the design and purpose of the study. One type consists of a narrative description and classification according to preestablished categories. The second type of analysis involves development of a guide to sort and categorize the data. The third type of analysis involves the interpretation of categorized data. Data may be coded and reconceptualized around central themes. The fourth type of analysis involves immersion and reflection in the narrative data to allow meaning to emerge from the data. Descriptive statistics may also be used to describe frequencies and distribution of data. Computerized analysis is available to assist with ethnographic coding and analysis.

Statistical Software

Statistical packages are available for data analysis. Factors to consider when selecting a statistical package are the types and power of tests that can be performed, the readability of results, graphic capability, ease of use, technical support, statistical advice, documentation, update capability, and cost. Commonly used statistical packages for nursing and the social sciences are SPSS, Systat, Statview, Minitab, Ethnograph, and data management and analysis through Excel or other software programs.

Results, Discussion, and Conclusion

Once the analyses are completed, the results are summarized and the hypotheses or research questions are answered. Then follows the discussion of the findings, in which the researcher explains the results and compares them with the theory or underlying framework for the study. In the conclusion phase of the study, the researcher formulates a succinct summary of results, examines limitations, and makes recommendations for practice. The generalizability of the study is discussed to determine if the results can be generalized to other settings and samples.

Dissemination of Results

Once the research study is complete, a report is prepared for the funding agency, for a thesis or dissertation, or for presentation or publication.

Components of a Research Report

A research report generally consists of an abstract, followed by a report of the study: the purpose and research questions; the design, methods, and procedures; the analyses and results; and the discussions, conclusions, and recommendations. The abstract consists of a 100- to 200-word description of the study: the purpose, framework, research question or hypothesis, sample, setting, design, procedure, results, conclusions, and recommendations.

The first part of the report includes the introduction, purpose, review of literature, framework for the study, need for the study, and research question or hypothesis. The introduction draws the reader's attention to the study. For example, a statistic related to the significance of the problem or a brief descriptive case situation may be cited. The *purpose* and significance of the problem are followed by a *review of literature*. The researcher selects and compares research findings, discusses relevant theory, and includes careful documentation of references. The review consists of a critical appraisal and summary of the literature, not a list of quotes or a list of studies. The review may precede or be preceded by a theoretical framework or model that guided the study. The need for the study is presented, along with the *research questions* or *hypotheses* tested.

The second part of the report discusses the *methods* and *procedures* used to obtain data. The sample is described with facts, such as gender, age, ethnicity, health status, or other attributes. The setting is a description of the agency, home, school, or other location; geographic area; urban or rural status; or other characteristics of the setting. The validity and reliability of the data collection instruments or the characteristics of the interview guide are described. The next section presents the data collection procedures, including human subjects' clearance (IRB approval), subject consent, and methods used to obtain data (eg, face-to-face or telephone interviews, questionnaires, mailed surveys). Qualitative research includes a description of entrée into the setting, the role of the researcher, and the interview or observation process.

The third section reports the *research findings,* which, for quantitative studies, are the results of the statistical analysis of the data, resulting in the answer to the research question or hypothesis testing. Tables, figures, or models may be used to explain or clarify the results. In qualitative analysis, the data are summarized, interpreted, and reported in narrative form. Tables and diagrams may be used to clarify results and describe themes; direct quotations may serve as exemplars.

The final section of the manuscript presents the *discussion, conclusions, and recommendations.* The discussion interprets and explains the research results and compares the results to other research findings. The conclusion summarizes the essence of the study and the limitations. A brief statement is made on the clinical implications of the findings, and specific recommendations are given as appropriate for research and practice.

A research report avoids jargon, is organized with headings, is brief, and is clearly written. The reference list includes all sources cited in the study and usually does not include personal communications and unpublished material. The report often includes biographical information on the researcher and a primary address for correspondence.

Submission of a Research Manuscript for Publication

A researcher may submit the report of the study to a journal for publication. First, the author needs to review journals to determine the best match for the article (eg, which journals publish clinical research, specialty research, or methodology pieces). The information for authors in the selected journals provides specific information on the format and submission process, including acceptance of unsolicited manuscripts.

COVER LETTER. The manuscript can be submitted with a cover letter to the editor, or a query letter can be sent to the editor of the journal without the manuscript to ask if the editor is interested in reviewing the manuscript for publication. In either case, the letter begins with a lead sentence or paragraph that captures the reader's interest. It is followed with a description of the article and why it would be of interest to the audience of the journal. The next section provides factual information about the research and highlights the author's credentials or other qualifications to write the article. The final paragraph offers a strong conclusion to convince the editor that the article should be published and then requests a response.

FACT SHEET. When the manuscript is submitted, it is accompanied by a fact sheet listing the the authors' names, their credentials and titles, and the address of one contact author for correspondence. The authors' names do not appear on any of the manuscript pages if the journal uses a blind peer review process.

MANUSCRIPT PARAMETERS. The manuscript should be clearly printed double spaced on quality 8 1/2 × 11 white paper with plain font and have at least 1-inch margins. The information for authors is followed for format, length, and reference format. Creative italics, bold print, or underlining are not recommended. Usually two to four copies are requested with pages numbered and without names. Tables are generally submitted camera ready, one per page, with site of insertion noted in the text.

When accepted, the author will be asked to assign rights to the manuscript to the journal. A biographical sketch and a disk copy of the manuscript are also submitted. The manuscript may be edited by the journal for style, spacing, and clarity. The author generally proofreads the galley copy for final approval.

Submission of an Abstract for a Presentation

A call for abstracts is a published invitation to researchers to submit an abstract describing their study for review for presentation at a conference. The presentation format may consist of the presentation of an individual research report or a presentation with other researchers in a symposium organized by topic. The format may also be in a visual poster or at a round table session. The call for abstracts is posted in advance of the conference by several months or more than a year to allow conference organizers time to select the abstracts for presentation, which is often done through a peer review process. The researcher then is invited to present and the conference brochures are printed with the list of presenters.

ABSTRACT FORMAT. The researcher prepares an abstract within the specified format. Often, the researcher must submit a camera-ready copy of the abstract formatted to fit a specified space. The abstract usually includes an informative title, the name and title of the researcher (unless there is a blind review process), and a brief summary of the purpose, sample, setting, methods, procedure, results, and conclusions. There is usually a general information sheet to be completed at the time of submission or when the abstract is accepted. The information includes preferred presentation format, needs for special equipment, and a brief biographical sketch, which will be used for introductions or printed in the proceedings of the conference.

PRESENTATION PARAMETERS. The presentation is often limited to 20 minutes, including time for questions. Generally there is a podium, microphone, and equipment for slides or overheads. The presenter may be responsible for forwarding the visuals, or assistance may be available. Practicing the presentation helps the presenter to stay within the time constraints and to coordinate the slides or other visual materials.

POSTER PRESENTATION. A poster presentation is generally scheduled for a specified time. The posters may be on display before or during the entire conference. The researcher usually stays near the poster during designated times to answer questions, discuss the findings, and exchange information with other conference participants.

Research Poster

A research poster is a brief summary of the study presented visually. The poster itself can vary from a self-produced display on poster board designed to stand or a manufactured poster backdrop, to a commercially produced computerized printout with specialized mounting. The contents include the title, author, sample, procedure, instruments, type of analysis, findings, major conclusions, and practice and research implications. The poster only presents the key points in phrases or diagrams with no details to deliver a clear message. Each of the sections is presented in outlined boxes of information. Tables, charts, or photographs may help clarify the study.

The printed lettering must be large enough to be read from several feet away to draw the attention of people passing by the poster. An effective poster is uncluttered, balanced, easy to read, and has visual appeal. Cost of materials includes quality paper, mounting boards, mounting materials, and background poster material. Software programs, such as Power-Point or Harvard Graphics, and a laser printer are useful. Graphic artists and printing services are available for a fee to assist with poster development, but an effective poster can be produced by the researcher.

Research Proposals

A research proposal is needed to obtain funding, approval from an IRB, approval from a thesis or dissertation committee, or to gain entrée into a research site. Development of a written logical, concise proposal also helps to refine the research design and avoid problems later.

A research proposal is a plan for a future study. The format and length varies according to the agency guidelines and purpose. For example, an IRB may restrict the proposal to a few pages and require limited review of literature, while a dissertation committee may require an extensive literature summary and critique.

The *proposal* begins with a convincing statement as to the importance of the research and a brief summary of the purpose of the planned research. A brief critical review of literature is presented, followed by the research questions or hypotheses. The design, methods, and procedures are presented in detail. Any risks to human subjects and plans for protection of human subjects are presented, including confidentiality, privacy, and informed consent. The sample, inclusion and exclusion criteria, and the setting are specified. The power analysis to support the sample size is included. The validity and reliability of the instrumentation and the plan for the analysis of data are detailed. The plan for evaluation and dissemination of results is also given. A time line specifies the timing of activities for accomplishment of each objective or phase of the research.

In a request for funding, a *budget* is also presented, which includes costs for personnel, consultation fees, statistical support, supplies, postage, telephone, computer equipment, software, instruments, duplicating, rentals, travel, and other direct costs associated with the research.

In-kind contributions, indirect costs, and foundation fees are also included. A budget justification is prepared to support the budget request.

Attachments to the proposal include copies of the consent, approval letters on letterhead from the agencies involved, all instruments that will be used to collect data, résumé or curriculum vitae of the researcher, approval from the institutional review board, and other letters of support or permission that may be required for the implementation of the study. Additional forms relative to affirmative action, declaration of a drug-free workplace, or other items may be required.

The format requirements vary, but all require a clear, organized, logical, easy-to-read presentation on quality paper. It is helpful to review examples of successful proposals.

Funding agencies include the National Institute for Nursing Research or other institutes, private foundations, voluntary agencies or professional groups with a research priority, university and hospital foundations, Sigma Theta Tau International, medical centers, pharmaceutical or medical supply companies, or numerous other agencies and individuals. The foundation offices in university settings can assist with searches for funding, and books and computer searches are available for obtaining information on funding sources.

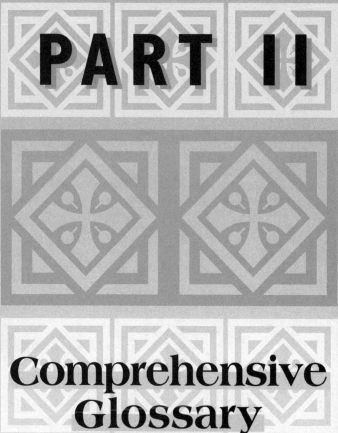

PART II

Comprehensive Glossary of Research Terms

A

α See alpha.

abscissa See X-axis.

absolute value The value of a number regardless of its positive or negative sign.

abstract A brief description of a research study providing a summary of the purpose, methods, and major results of the study. Usually appears at the beginning of a research report. Also called the research abstract.

accessible population The group of subjects available for a research study, often a nonrandom subset of the target population.

accidental sample A group of subjects most readily available or convenient for a research study.

acquiescence bias A tendency to respond affirmatively to all items on a self-report instrument, most often noted on social psychological data collection instruments. Also called acquiescence response set.

acquiescence response set See acquiescence bias.

active independent variable A variable that the investigator manipulates.

actors In qualitative research, people within a group of interest who are studied by the researchers, such as subjects from a particular cultural group who are studied by ethnographic researchers.

adjusted means The mean values of the dependent variables with adjustments made to remove the effects of co-variates.

adjusted R^2 The squared multiple correlation coefficient with an adjustment made for the number of predictors and sample size to improve the accuracy of the estimate.

after only design See post-test only design.

aim See purpose.

alpha (α) (1) The level of statistical significance designating the probability of committing a type I error. Also known as the p value. (2) A reliability coefficient, such as Cronbach's alpha, to estimate internal consistency.

alpha level The level of strength of statistical evidence necessary to determine the results of a study statistically significant.

alternate form reliability A determination of reliability of an instrument by administration of two or more forms of the same test to the same person at different times. The scores are compared to determine the relationship between the two forms. Also called parallel form reliability.

alternate form test A second form of a test used to establish reliability.

alternative hypothesis See hypothesis.

analysis The systematic organization and examination of data to determine the results of a study.

analysis of covariance (ANCOVA) A statistical procedure that allows the investigator to control for extraneous variables (covariates) while determining the effect of one or more treatments on the dependent measures.

analysis of variance (ANOVA) A statistical procedure that allows means of more than two groups to be compared simultaneously while maintaining control of the probability of type I error.

analytic induction A method used in qualitative research in which the researcher refines a theory by searching for negative cases and making refinements until no more negative cases are found.

anchors Specifications that define levels for a scale used to measure phenomena, usually presented at the beginning of the instrument or for each section of the instrument. Also the two extremes of an attribute stated at either end of the response set to an item measuring the attribute.

animal subjects Animals other than human that serve as participants in research.

anonymity The identity of the research subject remaining unknown and not linked with the information provided by the subject.

ANCOVA See analysis of covariance.

ANOVA See analysis of variance.

a priori A form of deductive reasoning in which theory and principles precede and influence research and systematic observation.

applied research Research intended to address specific practical problems and questions.

archives Public records or unpublished materials that serve as a primary source of information.

ARIMA See autoregressive integrated moving average.

array An assembly of data with scores arranged sequentially from lowest to highest.

assumptions (1) Beliefs or principles that are accepted as true based on logic or reason, without proof; may be implicit or explicit. (2) In statistics, the characteristics of the data that are believed to be true to perform a statistical procedure validly.

asymmetric distribution A distribution of values that is skewed and not evenly distributed over a normal curve.

attitude scale Self-report data collection instrument that asks the respondent to rate feelings or tendencies along a dimension.

attribute independent variable Preexisting characteristics of the subject, such as age or gender, that cannot be manipulated by the investigator but are observed and measured.

attrition A threat to the internal validity of a study caused by the loss of subjects participating in the research study.

auditability The ability of an independent researcher to follow the methodology, documentation of data, and conclusions of the original researcher.

authenticity Quality or state of being true and genuine, including truthful reporting in a primary source document.

autoregressive integrated moving average (ARIMA) A statistical procedure applied in the analysis of interrupted time series data.

axial coding A data analysis method used in grounded theory research to connect categories and subcategories through analysis of factors, such as conditions, contexts, interactions, or consequences, that link concepts.

axiom A summary of empirical support relating two concepts.

β See beta.

bar graph A graph to portray nominal or ordinal data with categories on the horizontal axis and frequencies on the vertical columns.

Bartlett's test of sphericity A statistical test used to examine whether the dependent variables are correlated in a MANOVA or canonical analysis.

baseline The measurement of a variable at the beginning of the study and before introduction of an experimental intervention.

basic research Research designed to expand the base of knowledge or to build theory for a discipline rather than to seek a solution for a problem. Also called pure research.

before–after design See pretest/post-test design.

beneficence The ethical principle to prevent harm to research subjects and to conduct research that will be of benefit.

beta (β) (1) Statistical testing term referring to the probability of making a type II error. (2) The standardized regression coefficient in the regression equation indicating the relative weights of the independent variables.

between-subjects design A research design in which two or more independent groups of subjects are compared, such as college graduates and high school graduates.

bias Any influence introduced by the researcher, subjects, instrumentation, data collection, or analysis of data that distorts the results of a study.

bimodal distribution A frequency distribution containing two modes that appear as two high-frequency peak values on a graphic display.

binomial distribution A probability distribution for a dichotomous variable.

biographical history A study of the life of a person in context of the period of time in which that person lived.

bivariate Consisting of two variables.

bivariate normal distribution A distribution of two variables in which scores on X are normally distributed for each value of Y, and scores on Y are normally distributed for each value of X.

bivariate regression A statistical procedure for obtaining a straight line to describe the relationship between two variables.

bivariate statistics Statistical procedures used to test the relationship between two variables.

blind review The review of a grant proposal or manuscript for publication or presentation that is conducted in a manner that the identities of the author and the reviewer remain unknown to one another in an attempt to reduce subjectivity in the review process.

blind study A study conducted using blind techniques in which either the experimenter in contact with subjects or the subjects are unaware of their assignment into the experimental or nonexperimental group. It can be single-blind if one is unaware or double-blind if both are unaware of the assignment.

blind techniques Procedures that are applied in experimental research in which the experimenters in contact with subjects or the subjects are unaware of whether they are receiving the experimental or nonexperimental intervention.

blocking An approach to control extraneous variables by changing the design to include them as independent variables.

borrowed theory A theory from one discipline applied to practice or research in another discipline.

Bonferroni adjustment/correction A statistical adjustment to reduce a significance level or increase a confidence level to correct for the problem created by multiple hypothesis testing; helps to reduce the problem of rejecting a false null hypothesis.

Box *M* test A statistical test to determine the homogeneity of a variance–covariance matrix.

bracketing A technique used in phenomenological research during which the researcher identifies judgments, preconceived ideas, personal biases, or knowledge about the phenomenon under study to suspend them and to specify how they may influence observations and conclusions.

broad-range theory See grand theory.

C

call for abstracts A request for submission of abstracts or summaries of research studies for consideration for presentation by the investigator at a research conference.

canonical analysis See canonical correlation.

canonical correlation A multivariate statistical procedure that examines the relationship between a set of two or more independent variables and a set of two or more dependent variables. Also called canonical analysis.

canonical correlation coefficient (R_c) In canonical analyses, the statistical term to express the relationship between pairs of composite variables.

card catalog Alphabetical listings of books by title, author, and subject.

carryover effect A confounding effect when a new treatment is introduced while the subject still experiences the effects of a previous treatment.

case-control study A research design in which a subject (case) with the condition of interest is compared with a subject (control) without the condition. This design is frequently used with retrospective studies to identify factors associated with certain conditions.

case study Type of research in which a single individual, group, institution, or situation is studied in depth to describe multiple dimensions of an experience.

category A classification of related concepts into a higher order, more abstract concept.

categorical variable A variable with discrete qualitative value, such as gender, eye color, or marital status.

categorizing A technique used in qualitative research to classify related concepts into a higher order broad concept.

causal direction A relationship between two variables in which changes in X result in changes in Y.

causal model A statistically tested model to explain the causes of a phenomenon.

causal modeling A process to develop and test a hypothetical model, which explains the causation of a phenomenon.

causal relationship A relationship between two variables in which the presence, absence, or amount of one variable (the cause) corresponds with the presence, absence, or amount of the second variable (the effect).

causal variable See independent variable.

causality The relating of causes to the resultant effects.

ceiling effect The effect of having scores at or near the highest value, decreasing the amount of variance and change.

cell One of the boxes in a table formed by the intersection of rows and columns.

central limit theorem The phenomenon in which the random sampling distribution of means tends to be normally distributed and becomes increasingly closer as the sample size increases.

central tendency A statistical index describing the clustering and distribution of scores. The most common measures are the mean, median, and mode.

chance error Random error through variation in results for a specified period of time, often unknown and unable to be controlled by the researcher.

change score The score obtained by subtracting the scores obtained at one point in time from the scores of the same variable obtained at a previous point in time.

checklist A format for written questionnaires in which the subject uses a check mark to indicate which items on a list are applicable.

chi-square goodness-of-fit test The test of fit of models used in statistical techniques, such as logistic regression and path analysis.

chi-square test of independence A nonparametric test of statistical significance with data measured at the nominal (categorical) level; compares the actual number in each group with the number expected by chance.

CINAHL See Cumulative Index of Nursing and Allied Health Literature.

class boundaries Points that set the limit for a group of scores in a frequency distribution. The points are midway between the highest score of one group and the lowest score of the next group.

class interval A group of scores in a frequency distribution.

class mark The midpoint in a group of scores in a frequency distribution located halfway between class boundaries.

clinical relevance The degree to which the purpose or findings of a study are applicable to or guide clinical practice.

clinical research Research studies that involve clients or have potential application to clinical practice.

clinical trial Experimental research testing the effectiveness of an intervention on a sample of human subjects.

closed-ended question A question in which the subject is forced to choose an answer from mutually exclusive alternatives.

cluster analysis A multivariate technique used with a group of subjects who are similar in certain characteristics or attributes to create homogeneous subsets. Individuals in each subset are more similar to each other than to individuals in other subsets.

cluster randomization Random assignment of certain groups of individuals to experimental treatment—useful when random assignment of individuals to different treatment groups is difficult.

cluster random sampling A probability sampling technique that involves repeated random sampling progressing from large to small units over two or more stages. An example is selection of samples from home health agencies, then selecting a sample of nurse case managers in home health agencies.

coding The process of data analysis used in grounded theory research in which observations are grouped and given an identification code for later analysis.

code of ethics The ethical principles established by the profession and society to guide research with human subjects. There are common principles across disciplines that are directed at beneficence, justice, and respect for human dignity in research.

codebook The directory that lists the kinds of data expected and the values and location of variables in a data set.

coefficient alpha See Cronbach's alpha.

coefficient of determination The proportion of variance (R^2) in the dependent variable explained by a group of independent variables included in the regression equation.

coercion of subjects The use of threats or rewards beyond the scope of research to persuade subjects to participate in a research study.

Cohen power test See power analysis.

cohort A group of subjects who share a common experience for a specific time.

cohort effect Changes in an individual that occur as a result of membership in a group of subjects under study.

cohort study A study of a group of individuals who share common characteristics or experiences for a specific time. Also called a prospective study.

collectively exhaustive categories Groupings or categories that are available for every possible response.

columns The vertical information in a table.

communality In factor analysis, a measure of the shared variance of a variable.

comparative study A descriptive research design that compares two or more groups who differ on the presence, absence, or value of the variable under study and are similar to one another in most other characteristics. The research may be conducted at one time or at multiple times.

comparison group A group of subjects whose scores on a dependent variable are used to evaluate the scores of the group under study when a control group is not part of the research design.

complex hypothesis A multivariate hypothesis that predicts the relationship between two or more independent variables and two or more dependent variables.

computer-assisted literature search A search of literature accomplished through a computer connected to a data base on a computer, a CD-ROM, or the internet. The search can be conducted by entering the topic, key words, titles, or authors' names.

concealment A situation involving collection of data in the natural setting without the informed consent of the human subjects under observation.

concept A symbolic representation of an abstract idea or phenomenon.

conceptual definition A statement of the general meaning of a concept or abstraction.

conceptual density Comprehensive, thorough data collection to the point that provides assurance that all possible findings have been generated regarding the phenomenon under investigation.

conceptually derived techniques Process of grouping data according to coding categories established by the researcher prior to data analysis.

conceptual framework In research, the interrelated concepts and ideas that guide research questions and the formulation of hypotheses for testing and establish a framework for integration of research findings. Also called a conceptual model.

conceptual literature Published or unpublished works related to conceptual or theoretical knowledge or professional issues. Also called theoretical literature.

conceptual map A diagrammatic display of the concepts or variables in a theory.

conceptual model See conceptual framework.

conceptual utilization Use of research results to expand knowledge and general thinking unrestricted by immediate practical application.

conclusion A brief summary of the research results at the end of a research report, usually including a statement relating results to the purpose of the study.

concurrent validity Test validity obtained by the correlation of results of two tests measuring the same concept administered to the subject at the same data collection time.

conditions The context or circumstances that may have an effect on the subject.

confidence interval The range of values estimated to contain the values for a population within a specified degree of probability.

confidence level The degree of probability that the values for a population occur within the confidence interval.

confidentiality Protection of the identity of human subjects and their individual responses from disclosure to the public.

confirmability A criterion to measure trustworthiness of a qualitative study that reflects credibility, auditability, and transferability of findings.

confirmatory factor analysis A factor analysis to confirm a hypothesized measurement model.

confounding variable A variable that is not the variable of interest in the research study but alters the relationship between the independent and dependent variables and affects the results of the study. The researcher attempts to control for extraneous variables in the design or with statistical procedures. Also known as an extraneous variable or intervening variable.

consensual validation The process of validation of an instrument through evaluation by a panel of experts.

consent form A written agreement signed by the subject explaining the study procedures, risks, benefits, and rights of the voluntary participant.

consistency A criterion that implies that the phenomenon occurs with the same meaning or behavior over time, that data are collected in the same manner from each subject at each point in time, or that terms and concepts have the same meaning when repeated over time.

consistency check A method to clean data and evaluate whether data entered at one point are compatible with data from the same subject entered at a second point.

constant comparative method A method used in grounded theory research in which newly acquired data and current data are continuously compared with one another to refine categories and themes.

constitutive definitions Explanation of a construct by description of other constructs and concepts.

construct An abstract phenomenon developed for scientific purposes, measured indirectly through study of less abstract indicators of the phenomenon.

construct validity The degree to which an instrument measures the construct it is intended to measure.

consumer An individual who reviews and uses research findings in education, research, or practice.

contact information Information obtained from subjects enrolled in longitudinal studies to enable them to be contacted at future data collection points. Such information might include home and work addresses for the subject, family, or friends who could assist in locating the subject.

contamination Accidental, undesirable mixing of treatment conditions.

content analysis (1) In qualitative research, the process of categorizing observations according to themes and concepts emerging from the data. (2) A method to make inferences based on systematic, objective, and statistical analyses of written text or oral communication and documentation. Also known as manifest content analysis.

content validity The degree that an instrument adequately samples the phenomenon under investigation.

context A set of properties or conditions that pertains to phenomena.

contingency table A table with cross-classification of data for two variables.

continuous variable A variable with no gaps between values along a dimension.

contract An award for funding given after approval of a proposal submitted by an investigator or group of investigators.

contrast effect A sequencing effect in an interview in which later responses are contrasted and compared with earlier responses.

control The process of holding constant extraneous influences that may have an effect on the dependent variable in a study. Also called research control.

control group In an experimental study, the group of subjects receiving standard care with no experimental treatment.

control condition Situation or condition used for comparison in an experimental study.

convenience sample A nonprobability sample of subjects readily available for participation in a study. Also called an accidental sample.

convenience sampling A nonprobability sampling procedure in which readily available individuals or groups are selected for participation in a study.

convergent validity A procedure to evaluate construct validity in which scores obtained with two measures of the same construct are compared for degree of correlation. High correlation indicates they are similar or convergent.

core category In grounded theory, the main concept that ties together all categories of data.

correlation A linear relationship between two variables that are at the ordinal, interval, or ratio level of measurement; variation in one variable is related to variation in the other variable and can be either positive or negative.

correlation coefficient A statistic that summarizes the degree and direction of the relationship between two variables, with scores ranging from +1 for a complete direct relationship to −1 for an inverse relationship, and a 0 to indicate no relationship.

correlation matrix A display of correlation coefficients for all combinations of relationships between two variables.

correlational research/studies A research design that explores the relationships between multiple variables measured at the same time without any active experimental treatment.

cost–benefit analysis A comparison of the cost of a project or risk of a treatment with the benefit to be gained.

counterbalancing A method to control for the effects of order by systematic variation in the order of treatments or items in a measurement scale.

covariance A measure of the degree of linear association of two variables.

covariate A variable that is controlled statistically or held constant while the effect of another variable is analyzed to determine more clearly the effect of the study variable and to limit the effect of extraneous variables.

cover letter A letter to a prospective research subject or reviewer to introduce a packet of materials.

covert data collection The collection of data in which the subject is unaware of the research process.

Cramer's V A measure to describe the magnitude of a relationship between nominal data when the contingency table is larger than four cells.

credibility A term to evaluate the truth and trustworthiness of findings in a qualitative study in which participants acknowledge that the findings reflect their experience.

criterion measure See criterion variable.

criterion-related validity The relationship between scores on a new measurement instrument and scores on an established standardized instrument for the same variable.

criterion variable The quality or level used to measure the effect of an independent variable. Also called criterion measure or dependent variable.

criterion referenced measure Measure used to determine whether an individual has achieved a desired effect.

critical incident technique A method in which subjects are asked to provide comprehensive information about a specific situation or phenomenon.

critical social theory The study of existing social problems to determine alternatives and promote responsibility.

critical region The area of values in a theoretical sampling distribution that are considered to be statistically significant. Also known as the region of rejection.

critical value The point in the sampling distribution at which the values are considered to be statistically significant.

critique An objective, critical, scientific evaluation of a research report for quality and for potential contribution to knowledge or practice.

Cronbach's alpha A commonly used indicator of internal consistency reliability or homogeneity of a measure in which each item within the scale is correlated with other items simultaneously.

crossover design An experimental design in which an individual or group of individuals is assigned to both the experimental treatment and the control conditions or to multiple treatments in random order.

cross-sectional study A research design in which one section of the population is sampled at one time. The sample includes broad representation of people with characteristics of interest, such as age, development, time since diagnosis, or other factors, to allow the researcher to make inferences about trends over time.

cross-tabulation A procedure to determine the number of cases when two or more variables are considered at a time; usually presented in a table with cells representing each of the possibilities.

cross-validation The process of validating findings by comparing the analysis conducted with one subset of the sample to a replication analysis conducted with another subset.

cues Hints, suggestions, or indicators used in an interview that may initiate a response or suggest a direction or idea.

cultural scene A term to indicate the people, objects, and behaviors in a social scene.

Cumulative Index to Nursing and Allied Health Literature (CINAHL) A computerized (CD-ROM or on-line) or print data base listing nursing and allied health literature.

cumulative frequency The number of observations in a specified interval or any preceding interval.

cumulative scale A scale constructed with items arranged in order of increasing intensity so that agreement at one level includes agreement with all previous levels. See Guttman scale.

curvilinear An association between two variables in which a curved line best fits the relationship.

cyclical variability Variation in a phenomenon that occurs in repeated patterns over time.

D

data Pieces of information and facts systematically collected during a research study; the plural of datum.

data analysis The systematic organization, examination, and manipulation of data to answer the research question or test the hypothesis of the study.

data base The set of information obtained during a study and arranged in an organized, systematic fashion to allow retrieval and analysis.

data-based literature Reports of completed research studies. Also known as empirical literature, research, or scientific literature.

data cleaning The process of organizing and checking data for completion and accuracy in recording or data entry before proceeding to analysis.

data collection The process of gathering information relevant to the purpose of the study.

data display Organized presentation of qualitative data in preparation for analysis and conclusions.

data entry The process of entering data into the computer to create a data base for analysis.

data matrix Organization of data into rows and columns, usually with cases in rows and values for variables in columns.

data modification See data transformation.

data reduction The process of synthesizing information from multiple variables into a smaller number of variables to facilitate data analysis and reporting.

data saturation See saturation.

data transformation The process of organizing and recoding information in the data base to prepare it for data analysis.

debriefing Meeting with research subjects at the conclusion of their participation to discuss the research study.

deception The act of providing false information or withholding information from subjects when such knowledge might influence their responses.

deductive reasoning The logical thought process of moving from generalizations to specific conclusions, or from theory to specific observations.

definition of terms Description of terminology to explain language used in a study.

degrees of freedom (df) The statistical term used in determining statistical significance, which indicates the number of values that are free to vary and is a function of the number in the sample.

delimitation Characteristics that limit the sample to a homogenous population.

Delphi technique A technique to obtain consensus from a panel of experts who give individual feedback on a subject that is then judged by the entire panel. The process is repeated, building on information obtained in each round, until some agreement is obtained.

demographic information See demographic variable.

demographic question A question to obtain information to describe the subject, such as age, gender, socioeconomic status, or other descriptive characteristics.

demographic variable Characteristics that describe the subjects, such as age, gender, marital status, educational level, or other attribute.

dependent *t*-test A form of statistical *t*-test used when one set of scores is dependent on another set of scores.

dependability See stability reliability.

dependent variable The effect achieved by the independent variable or the experimental treatment. Also called the criterion variable.

descriptive research Nonexperimental research studies conducted to describe phenomena or to study relationships between variables without any attempt to experiment or manipulate variables.

descriptive statistics Statistics used to describe, explain, and summarize numerical data.

descriptive theory Theory that describes a phenomenon, event, situation, or relationship, including the composition and situational context.

determinism The belief that phenomena have causes and do not randomly occur.

deviation score A score obtained by subtracting an individual score from the mean score of the distribution.

design The plan for a research study, which includes the setting, sample, methods, procedures, and analytical procedures to be used in the study.

dichotomous variable A variable that has only two values, such as gender.

dichotomous scale A measurement instrument that provides only two categories, such as "yes" or "no."

differential selection Systematic differences in the assignment of subjects to treatment or control conditions.

direct costs Costs associated with a project, such as salaries or supplies.

direct effect The effect of an independent variable on a dependent variable; a direct path in a causal model.

direct relationship An association in which a cause results in an effect.

directional hypothesis A hypothesis that predicts the direction of the relationship between the independent and dependent variables. The hypothesis uses only one tail of the distribution in determining the value needed to reject the null hypothesis. Also known as a one-tailed hypothesis.

discriminant function analysis A multivariate statistical procedure used to predict a dependent variable measured on the nominal scale, such as a categorical group. The independent variables can be interval or ratio level data or dichotomous nominal data.

discriminant validity A method to validate a construct by differentiating the construct under study from other similar constructs. One instrument is used to measure two different constructs to produce different results.

discussion The section of the research report that discusses and explains the results of the data analysis and hypothesis testing.

disproportionate sampling design A sampling strategy in which the researcher selects members of different strata in the population in larger proportions than found in the population. The purpose is to ensure representation in the sample of individuals from different strata. Also known as disproportionate stratified sampling.

disproportionate stratified sampling See disproportionate sampling design.

distribution A term used to describe the magnitude and spread of obtained scores or values.

distribution free statistics See nonparametric statistics.

divergent validity A method to validate a construct by comparing scores obtained with two instruments, one to test the construct and the other to test an opposite construct. The scores are expected to have a negative relationship.

double-blind study A research study in which neither the researcher nor the subjects know which subjects are in the experimental group or in the control group.

double-barreled question A question that asks two questions simultaneously, requiring more than one answer.

drift The tendency to code differently over time.

dummy variable Dichotomous variables with the values of 0 and 1 created for statistical analysis.

effect coding A method used to code categorical variables for multivariate analysis with 1, 0, and −1.

effect size A statistical term to indicate the magnitude of the results as small, moderate, or large for the phenomenon of interest. The phenomenon may be a relationship between two variables, the difference between groups, or the degree to which the variable is found in the population.

eigenvalue A statistical term used in factor analysis that is the sum of the squared weights for each factor.

electronic data base Bibliographic files available for literature searches through a computer, either on-line or with compact disks.

element The most basic member of a population.

eligibility criteria The selection criteria used by the researcher to include or exclude subjects in the research sample.

embodiment In phenomenology, the consciousness or awareness of the world and ability to access the world through the body; an individual perceiving and being in the world through the mind and body.

emergent design In a qualitative study, a design that develops as the study progresses according to the knowledge obtained.

emic perspective In ethnographic research, the understanding of the culture, including language, beliefs, experiences and world view, as seen by the natives of the culture (insider's view).

empirical data Objective evidence or data collected through one of the senses. Also known as empirical evidence.

empirical evidence See empirical data.

empirical generalization A statement about the nature of phenomena based on data presented from several research studies.

empirical indicators The evidence obtained about a phenomenon that connects it with other concepts in the real world.

empirical literature See data-based literature.

empirical precision The requirement that concepts within a theory be related to observable reality.

empirical theory Theory based on objective, scientific evidence that can be tested. The theory is used to describe, explain, and predict the objective world.

empirical research Research studies that focus on objective scientific methodology and collection of data to form or test theory.

empirics Knowledge organized into theories and laws about the objective world.

endogenous variable In path analysis, a variable that varies according to other variables in the model.

entrée The process of gaining access to subjects and cooperation for conducting a qualitative research study.

epidemiology The study of health and deviations from health in populations. The studies include descriptive, analytical, and experimental research to analyze patterns of health and determine causality of disease and illness.

epistemic definition See operational definition.

epistemology In philosophy, the study of the history, limits, and validity of knowledge.

equimax method A statistical rotational technique used in factor analysis to simplify factors and variables.

equivalence The degree of similarity between two or more alternate forms of a measurement instrument.

error of measurement The difference between obtained scores and true scores. Also known as error variance.

error variance See error of measurement.

essences In qualitative studies, facets related to the ideal or the true meaning of phenomena that facilitate common understanding of the phenomena.

estimation The use of values obtained in a sample to estimate or infer the value in the population.

eta A correlation ratio of a linear or nonlinear relationship between nominal or continuous variables.

eta squared In ANOVA, the statistic that indicates the degree of variance in the dependent variable explained by the independent variables.

ethics The moral values and professional code that guide research conduct and protect human subjects. Also called research ethics.

ethnographic study A descriptive research study of a culture or subculture using ethnographic methodology.

ethnography The detailed study of a cultural group that describes and interprets their cultural patterns and world view.

ethnomethodology The method of researching a cultural group or subculture in which a researcher becomes part of the culture to conduct fieldwork and collects and analyzes information in the context of the culture.

ethnonursing research The study of the culture's perspectives, beliefs, and practices related to nursing care and health.

etic perspective In ethnographic research, an outsider's view and interpretation of the world view of a group.

evaluation research The use of scientific objective methods to judge the quality or value of a program, treatment, practice, policy, or other process.

event sampling A sampling method in which behaviors or other factors are observed during a specific event.

event-triggered observations A method of research in which data collection is initiated by the occurrence of an event or behavior.

exemplars The use of key narrative phrases or brief stories that exemplify and capture the essence of a concept or phenomenon of concern.

exogenous variable In path analysis, a variable that is determined by factors external to the model.

experiment Scientific studies in which the investigator randomly assigns subjects to experimental or nonexperimental (control) conditions, manipulates the cause (independent variable), and measures the effect on the dependent variable of interest.

experimenter bias/effect A threat to the external validity of a study that occurs when the researcher has an unintended effect on the subjects.

experimental design A scientific research design to test an experimental hypothesis using random assignment of subjects to groups, an experimental treatment, and a control group.

experimental group The subjects who receive the experimental treatment, conditions, or intervention in an experimental study. Also known as the treatment group.

experimental hypothesis In an experimental study, a statement of the predicted relationship between the independent (treatment) variable and the dependent variable. Also known as the alternative hypothesis.

experimental intervention See experimental treatment.

experimental research A scientific research study to test an experimental hypothesis characterized by random assignment of subjects into research groups, a treatment in which the researcher manipulates a variable or condition, and use of a control group that does not receive the experimental treatment.

experimental treatment The experiment, intervention, or condition being manipulated by the researcher in an experimental study. Also called an experimental intervention, intervention, or treatment.

experimental variance The amount of variance in the dependent variable attributable to the experimental treatment (independent variable).

expert A person with knowledge or experience with the phenomenon of interest who evaluates or helps develop research instruments, design, analysis, or other aspects of a research study.

expert panel A group of experts who assist with the evaluation or development of research instruments, design, analysis, or other aspects of a research study. Also called a panel of experts.

explanatory study Research study that seeks to explain causal relationships, generally consisting of experimental studies.

explanatory theory A logical explanation of causal relationships about phenomena.

exploratory factor analysis   See factor analysis.

exploratory research   (1) Research studies that are conducted on phenomena that are relatively unknown. (2) Preliminary or pilot studies to test instruments or methods.

ex post facto   After the fact or event has taken place.

ex post facto research   Nonexperimental research that takes place after the event or after variation in the independent variable has occurred.

external criticism   The process of judging the authenticity or genuineness of primary sources in historical research.

external validity   The ability to generalize the findings of one study to another sample, setting, or population.

extraneous variable   See confounding variable.

extraneous variance   The amount of variance in the dependent variable caused by factors other than the independent variables.

extreme response set   A bias in self-report instruments in which the subjects select the extreme responses to each item.

F

F ratio   A statistic to test the null hypotheses in ANOVA based on comparison of the variation between groups with the variation within groups. If the between-group variation is large relative to the within-group variation, the F ratio will be large and there could be a significant difference between groups.

F test   See F ratio.

face validity A subjective evaluation of a measurement instrument that determines that it measures what it intends to measure based on the way it appears (the "face" of it).

fact An idea or thing accepted as being true.

factor A characteristic with which to classify and group observations or variables.

factor analysis A statistical procedure that is used to explore concepts, build theory, or confirm and test hypotheses about constructs. It can be used to analyze multiple variables or items and group them into a smaller number of variables according to common characteristics called factors. It is also a method to examine which items in a set of items about a construct of interest measure similar or different characteristics of the construct. For example, in testing an instrument, if similar items covary in a similar fashion, they are grouped into a factor that can be named by the researcher according to the underlying characteristic that grouped them together.

factor extraction The first phase of factor analysis in which the correlation matrix of variables is analyzed to identify clusters of highly correlated variables and to reduce the number of factors.

factor loading In factor analysis of an instrument, the weight that represents the degree to which an item in the instrument loads on a factor or is similar to the characteristics measured by the factor.

factor matrix In factor analysis, a correlation matrix between every variable and the factor.

factor rotation The phase of factor analysis in which the clusters of highly correlated variables are statistically manipulated to cluster items further on a factor.

factorial design An experimental design in which two or more independent variables are manipulated and analyzed to determine the main effect and possible interaction effects of the independent variables.

feasibility An evaluation of the costs and benefits of a study, including availability of resources, personnel, time, access, and other factors that affect the possibility of conducting a research study.

feminist inquiry The study of problems related to women or from a woman's perspective.

field experiment An experiment conducted in a natural setting instead of a laboratory setting.

field notes Notes written by a qualitative researcher in the field situation to record observations about people, objects, places, behaviors, or events. Also known as observational notes.

field research Research method involving data collection in the naturalistic or real life setting ("in the field").

filler questions Questions used to distract the subject from the content or purpose of the research questions to change the pattern or to help the subject rest between focused questions.

findings The results of a study.

Fisher's exact test A statistical procedure to test the significance of the difference in proportions when the sample size is small or cells in the contingency table contain no values.

fittingness See transferability.

fixed-alternative question A question that offers a specified set of responses from which the subject must select the response that is most appropriate.

floor effect The effect of having scores at or near the lowest possible value, which reduces variability and measurement of change in the variable.

focused interview   An interview guided by general questions about the topic of interest.

focus group   A group of individuals gathered to discuss, provide expertise or information about, or work on a selected topic.

follow-up study   A study of individuals who have experienced a condition or variable of research interest in the past.

forward stepwise multiple regression analysis   See stepwise multiple regression analysis.

formative evaluation research   Research conducted at the beginning or during the implementation of a program or intervention. The purpose is to evaluate and improve quality and effectiveness during the implementation of the program.

frame of reference   Knowledge, experience, and attitudes affecting one's perception and perspective of the world.

framework   The theoretical or conceptual basis for a research study.

frequency count   The listing or counting of the number of observations of nominal or ordinal level data in a selected category.

frequency distribution   A descriptive statistical method of summarizing all the scores and frequency of occurrence for each score in a data set, displayed in order by the value of the score.

frequency polygon   A graphic presentation using dots and connecting lines to represent the frequency distribution of interval or ratio data in a research report.

Friedman test   A nonparametric statistical test for analyzing differences in paired groups or with repeated measures studies with a single sample.

full disclosure   The provision of complete information to research subjects about the purpose of the study, procedures, risks and benefits, and rights for subjects.

functional relationship   A relationship or association between two variables in which a variation in one is associated with a variation in the other.

futuristic design   Descriptive research design in which the researcher observes antecedent and consequent variables as they naturally occur.

galley proofs   Papers with the typeset format for an article, book, or other printed material to be published.

gamma   Nonparametric statistic to measure association.

Gantt chart   A schedule of activities for a research study that highlights the sequencing and relationships of research activities.

Gaussian curve   See normal distribution.

generalizations   A summary of empirical or theoretical observations about phenomena.

generalizability   The inference that the findings of a study represent phenomena in the population beyond the study sample or the degree to which the findings are generalizable.

generational effect   Effect of being born and raised within a specific time period.

genuine   A finding that a primary source is authentic and a true source of data.

goodness of fit   A statistic to compare the observed probabilities with the predicted probabilities in a statistical model.

grand mean In an ANOVA, the mean for all the observations from all of the groups.

grand theory A theory that encompasses the entire domain of the discipline and, as such, cannot be tested in its entirety by traditional empirical methods. Also called a broad-range theory or macrotheory.

grand tour question General opening question that presents an overview or preview of the topic to be discussed.

grant Funding for a proposal that enables researchers to conduct a project.

grantsmanship The art of being able to write a research proposal successfully and receive financial support for the study.

grant proposal A research proposal that includes a budget, an outline of the entire research project, and a summary of the qualifications of the researcher, which is then submitted to an agency for consideration for funding.

graph A pictorial display to describe and compare research data.

graphic rating scale A scale in which subjects are asked to rate a factor or attribute along a continuum, anchored by words such as "strongly disagree" to "strongly agree."

grounded theory Theory that is constructed from theoretical propositions based on data obtained in the real world.

grounded theory method An inductive approach to research using systematic observations in the natural world to build theory.

grounded theory research A type of study in which qualitative data are collected and analyzed to build theoretical propositions and theory that are based ("grounded") in real-world observations about social psychological and social structural processes.

guessing tendency   The tendency to select an answer on a questionnaire whether or not the respondent is sure of an answer.

Guttman scale   Format for a measurement instrument in which agreement with a higher level response indicates agreement with all levels below the selected response. Also known as cumulative scale.

halo effect   A type of response bias in which an attitude or trait influences the subject to respond in the same fashion to every item on the topic. For example, the subject may respond positively or negatively to every question related to a sensitive topic.

Hawthorne effect   A threat to the external validity of a research study in which the subject's awareness of being in the research study alters his or her responses.

hermeneutics   A qualitative research design closely related to phenomenology in which the researcher studies the lived experiences of people to understand the meaning and context of the experiences.

heterogeneity   A situation in which the sample composition or conditions are dissimilar or have wide variation on a measure.

heterogeneous sample   A sample in which the subjects are dissimilar on some characteristic.

heteroscedasticity   A property of variance of two variables in which for each value of X, the variablity of Y differs.

hierarchical multiple regression analysis A statistical procedure for analyzing the effect of multiple independent variables on a dependent variable. The researcher enters the variables into the regression according to a predetermined order based on the purpose and logic of the study.

histogram A graphic representation of the frequency distribution of interval or ratio data.

historical research Systematic research studies of the past using historical research methodology.

historical research method The systematic method of collecting, analyzing, and interpreting data about people, events, or phenomena that occurred in the past.

historian/historiographer One who studies or writes about history or conducts historical research.

history threat A threat to the internal validity of a study in which simultaneous external events occur outside the research study that can affect the dependent variable.

holistic analysis An evaluation of a research study for logical consistency between the parts of the study.

homogeneity (1) The degree to which items in an instrument consistently measure the same characteristic. Also known as internal consistency reliability. (2) The degree to which objects, subjects, or variables are similar or have low variation on a measure.

homogeneous sample The degree to which the research subjects are similar on some characteristic.

homoscedasticity A property of variance of two variables in which for each value of X, the variablity of Y is about the same.

human subjects review board See institutional review board.

hypothesis A statement of the predicted relationship between two or more variables in a study. Also called the alternative hypothesis.

hypothesis testing A technique in inferential statistics to test the null hypothesis in a sampling distribution.

hypothesis-testing validity An approach to establishing construct validity of a measurement instrument. The theory underlying the instrument's design is used to develop hypotheses for testing based on a range of scores on the instrument. The hypotheses are tested and results analyzed to determine whether they confirm the expected relationships.

immersion A term used in qualitative research to describe the degree to which the researcher is engaged or absorbed in the detailed analysis, synthesis, and description of data.

impact analysis An evaluation of the effect of a program or intervention on the outcome, without use of an experimental design to control other effects. Also called an outcome analysis.

implementation The ability to apply an intervention or condition into practice.

incidence The number of new cases of a disease or other condition in a specified population during a particular time.

incremental intervention A treatment administered in varying amounts over time.

independent samples An experimental research design in which subjects are randomly assigned to one of two or more treatment groups.

independent *t*-test See *t*-test.

independent variable The intervention, treatment, or condition that is manipulated by the researcher in an experimental study. Also called the treatment, causal, or predictor variable.

indexes Reference materials that provide information on books and journals by title, author, or subject.

indirect costs The overhead or institutional costs separate from the direct costs of the study, which are incorporated into a research budget.

indirect effect The effect of an independent variable on a dependent variable that occurs through a mediating variable. An indirect path in a causal model.

indirect observation Inferences made about a concept that cannot be directly observed; inferences based on objective data made with indirect measures of the concept.

indirect relationship A causal association in which a third variable causes or affects the relationship between two variables.

inductive theory building The process of developing theory by making generalizations based on specific observations.

inductive reasoning The logical thought process of moving from specific observations to general conclusions.

inferential statistics Statistics used to make conclusions and inferences about the probability of the findings observed in a sample also occurring in a larger population.

informant The individual who provides information or data about a phenomenon to the researcher in a qualitative study.

informant checking In a qualitative study, asking an informant to verify a researcher's findings.

informed consent A subject's agreement to participate in a research study after receiving information on voluntary participation, study procedures, and risks and benefits of the study.

input evaluation In evaluation research, an assessment of the ability of the people involved to carry out the program, strategies for achievement of the outcomes, and implementation methods.

institutional review board (IRB) A group of people in an agency who review proposed and ongoing research studies involving human subjects. Their purpose is to evaluate risks to human subjects and determine whether the research is ethical, including aspects such as use of informed consent, voluntary subjects, and confidentiality. Also called human subjects review board.

instruments Tools or devices the researcher uses to measure phenomena in a research study, such as a questionnaire, survey, interview guide, thermometer, or scale. Also called research instruments or research tools.

instrumental utilization Application of research findings to practice.

instrumentation change See instrumentation threat.

instrumentation system In physiological research, the entire set of measurement devices used to collect and record data.

instrumentation threat A threat to the internal validity of a study due to inaccuracy of the measurement device, inaccurate recording, reaction to the instrument, or changing the instrument used to obtain data between two collection points. These factors, rather than the experimental treatment, account for part of the effect on the dependent variable.

intellectual history A qualitative study of the ideas and attitudes of an individual, group, or time in history.

intentionality In phenomenology, the belief that consciousness is consciousness of something and that interior perception works with exterior perception. For example, one cannot see without seeing something.

interaction effect Two or more independent variables acting in combination to have an effect on the dependent variable, rather than acting as two separate variables.

intercoder reliability See inter-rater reliability.

internal consistency The degree to which items in a measurement scale measure the same concept or attribute. Also called internal consistency reliability or homogeneity.

internal criticism In historical research, an evaluation of the reliability, authenticity, and consistency of historical data.

internal validity The degree to which the independent variable (treatment), not extraneous variables, accounts for the effect on the dependent variable.

interobserver reliability See inter-rater reliability.

interpretation The process of explanation or determination of the meaning of a phenomenon.

interquartile range The portion of values in the middle half (50%) of a frequency distribution.

inter-rater reliability The degree to which two independent observers agree on the rating of observations or coding of qualitative data. Also called intercoder reliability or interobserver reliability.

interrelationship studies Nonexperimental research studies that measure associations, such as correlational, ex post facto, predictive, and developmental studies.

interrupted time series Experimental intervention inserted at a point in a series of observations.

interval data   Data that can be categorized and ordered by ranks on a scale with equal distances between ranks with an arbitrary 0, such as temperature.

interval measure   Measurement that obtains interval level data.

interval estimation   A statistical procedure that enables the researcher to calculate the range of values expected to contain the values for the population.

interval scale   A level of measurement used to indicate the rank order of magnitude and equal magnitudes of difference along a dimension. A given interval represents the same difference between any two points along the scale. Examples include temperature and time.

intervening variable   See confounding variable.

intervention   The experimental treatment or conditions manipulated by the researcher in an experimental study. Also the structure of the research setting.

interview   A method of data collection in which the researcher asks questions to obtain information from the participant. The researcher may use a written guide or follow a protocol for questions and may conduct the interview session face to face or over the telephone.

interview schedule   A research data collection instrument that contains directions, questions, and space for responses.

intuiting   In qualitative research, thinking through the data and analysis to achieve true comprehension and accurate interpretation of the meaning in the data.

inverse relationship   See negative relationship.

ipsative control   Research technique in a repeated measures design in which the subject serves as his or her own control. The values at baseline are compared with values obtained over time.

irregular variability Variation in a time series design with an uneven pattern related to unknown causes.

isomorphism In measurement theory, the similarity between the measures of an instrument and reality.

item A single question on a questionnaire or measurement scale.

item reversal Reversing the direction of the scoring on certain items in an instrument.

item-total correlation An evaluation of internal consistency reliability of an instrument that measures one concept. The degree that each item is correlated with the total score for the instrument indicates internal consistency.

iteration A repetition, as in repeated analyses of matrices in factor analysis.

journal club A group that meets to discuss or critique published research articles for personal education and for evaluation of applicability to education, research, or practice.

judgmental sample See purposive sample.

justice The ethical principle that states that human subjects are to be treated fairly.

Kendall's tau A nonparametric correlation coefficient used to indicate the magnitude of the relationship between variables measured at the categorical or ordinal level of measurement.

key informant A person who has special knowledge about the phenomenon or status in the group and is willing to participate in a research study.

knowledge A body of information, facts, or perceptions accepted as true.

known groups technique A technique to validate the construct of an instrument by using it to test selected groups who are predicted to achieve different scores based on the theory underlying the instrument. The obtained scores are compared with the predicted scores.

Kruskal-Wallis test A nonparametric test with ordinal data (rank ordered scores) to compare three or more independent populations.

Kuder-Richardson (KR-20) coefficient The estimate for internal consistency reliability (homogeneity) of an instrument with a set of dichotomous response items.

kurtosis The peakness or flatness of a distribution.

laboratory study Research conducted in a special setting created and controlled by the researcher.

law A theory with sufficient objective scientific evidence to be accepted as truth.

latency A time lapse between the treatment and the response or resulting behavior.

latent content analysis A method to study qualitative data in which each portion of text is considered in context of the entire text.

latent variable A confounding effect caused by a treatment variable activating a response from a prior treatment.

learning effect A confounding effect caused by the subject's response to the pattern of repetition of the treatment, rather than the treatment itself.

least-squares estimation Statistical estimate that minimizes the sums of squares of error terms. Also called the ordinary least squares.

leptokurtotic distribution A distribution with a pronounced sharp peak.

level of measurement One of four categories of measurement according to the nature of the data and the statistical analyses that are able to be performed: nominal, ordinal, interval, and ratio.

level of significance The probability of rejecting a null hypothesis when it is true (type I error). The level (commonly .05 or .01) is established prior to data analysis, and symbolized by a or p. Also called the probability level.

life context The matrix of personal and environmental interactions that takes place over a lifetime.

life history A qualitative research method in which the researcher listens to the life story of an individual or group of people who have an experience of interest to the researcher. The intent is to gain insight into the reality of the experience.

life table analysis A statistical method used when the dependent variable is a time interval between the onset and termination of an event. Also called survival analysis.

Likert scale An instrument to measure attitude with a series of items. There are usually five to seven responses to each item, which range from strongly agree to strongly disagree. Also called summated rating scale.

limitation The weaknesses and uncontrolled variables affecting a study.

linearity In instrumentation, the degree to which the variation of the output of an instrument follows variation in the input.

linear regression A statistical procedure in which variation in one variable predicts variation in the other variable, which can be described as a straight line.

linear structural relations analysis (LISREL) A statistical multivariate technique used to test a causal model to explain the causes of phenomena.

line graph The relationship between two variables graphically displayed with a line to connect the values.

LISREL See linear structural relations analysis.

listwise deletion A strategy to delete cases with missing data from a data base.

literature controls A situation in which data about subjects from published studies serve as data for a study.

literature review A critical analysis of research related to the topic or purpose of the study to identify knowledge gaps, gain insight into research design and methods for the topic, and gain a context for the problem and results of the study.

lived experience In phenomenological studies, a concept that refers to living through, rather than thinking about, experiences and conditions.

local theory A theory that applies only to the sample population and is not generalizable to the larger population.

log In participant observation research, the record of observations of people, events, and other phenomena that occur during the study.

logical positivism The philosophical roots of scientific methods.

logistic regression   A statistical multivariate technique to analyze the relationships between multiple independent variables and a dependent variable that is measured at the nominal level. Also called logit analysis.

logit analysis   See logistic regression.

longitudinal study   A nonexperimental research study with data collection from the same sample at repeated points in time.

macrotheory   See grand theory.

magnitude estimation   A method to measure the degree or strength of a phenomenon by asking respondents to mark corresponding numbers on a line with numbers or other indicators of variation from low or none to high or all.

main effects   The effects of a single independent variable on the dependent variable in a study with multiple independent variables.

mailed survey   A self-report survey instrument that is returned to the researcher by mail.

manifest content analysis   See content analysis.

manipulation   The introduction or addition of an independent variable (treatment, intervention, change) by the researcher in an experimental or quasi-experimental study to observe the effect on the dependent variable.

manipulation check   A follow-up test to verify whether the experimental manipulation was effectively implemented.

Mann-Whitney U test   A nonparametric statistical procedure to test whether there is a difference between two independent populations based on the distribution of ranked-level data.

MANOVA See multivariate analysis of variance.

MANCOVA See multivariate analysis of covariance.

matching The pairing of subjects designed to control confounding variance. Each subject in the experimental group is matched with a subject in the control group based on similarity on one or more variables. Also called pair-matching.

maturation threat A threat to the internal validity of a study that results when changes in the outcome measure (dependent variable) occur as the subjects age.

matrix (1) In qualitative research, a display of qualitative data with an arrangement of clusters of descriptive data around an event or experience. (2) A display of relationships between continuous variables in quantitative research (see correlation matrix).

maximum likelihood estimation A statistical estimate of the parameter values most likely to have generated the observed data.

McNemar test A statistical procedure to test the difference for two paired (nonindependent) population proportions.

mean A measure of central tendency; the descriptive statistic that is the arithmetic average of the observations.

meaning adequacy The degree of agreement between the operational definition, or meaning of a concept, and the indicators used to measure the concept.

measurement The assignment of specified numerical values to an amount of some attribute of an event or object.

measurement norms The values obtained when using a measure, such as the mean or standard deviation.

measure of central tendency The number that is the central value or most typical value around which data are grouped.

measure of variability The degree that observations vary in a distribution of values.

measures of relationship Statistics that present the association or correlation between variables.

measures to condense data Statistical procedures to reduce and summarize data.

median (Md, Mdn) The middle number in a set of observations; half of the observations are above the number, and half are below.

median test A statistical test to compare the difference in medians between two groups.

mediating variable A variable that affects the relationship between two other variables.

member check A method to validate qualitative data through discussion with people knowledgeable about the event.

meta analysis A statistical method to synthesize the findings of multiple quantitative studies on a specific topic by analyzing the size of the effect of the independent variable on the dependent variable.

metatheory Theory formulated about theory, such as theories about the development or categorization of theory.

methodological notes In naturalistic studies, notations made about the methods used to obtain data.

methodological research A scientific study of the instruments and strategies used to collect and analyze data.

methods The procedures and strategies used in a research study to obtain and analyze data. Also called research methods.

microtheory A theory that is focused on a specific phenomenon, is often situation specific, and can be tested, but it may not be generalizable to other situations.

middle-range theory A testable theory focused on a specific phenomenon, which includes several interrelated concepts believed to describe, explain, or predict phenomena.

minimal risk Research risk in which the risk to participants is anticipated to be no more than the amount of risk experienced in routine daily life.

missing values Observations missing in a set of data for a subject due to omitted responses or incomplete data entry.

mixed results Research findings that partially support and partially do not support the research hypothesis.

modality A description of the number of peaks in the distribution values.

modal class The category with the greatest number of observations of nominal and ordinal level data.

mode (Mo) The most frequently occurring value or category in a set of data; a measure of central tendency.

model A symbolic representation used to demonstrate the interrelationships among a set of concepts or phenomena.

molar approach A method to study behavior in which large groups of behavior are analyzed and treated as a whole.

molecular approach A method to study behavior in which small specific behaviors are the unit of observation and analysis.

monotonic relationship Correlation in which there is a consistent direction and degree of association between X and Y throughout all the values.

mortality threat The loss of participants in a study, which poses a threat to the internal validity of the study, especially if there is a great difference in the drop-out rate between the experimental and control groups.

multicollinearity Interrelatedness of the independent variables, which creates problems in the analysis of data and evaluation of results.

multimethod research Research in which multiple methods are used to analyze a phenomenon of concern. The methods can include both qualitative and quantitative approaches to data collection and analysis of the same phenomenon.

multimodal distribution A frequency distribution containing more than one mode that appears as more than one high frequency peak on a graphic display.

multiple case design The use of two or more cases in a case study research project.

multiple choice Questionnaire format in which the subject must choose from several response options.

multiple classification analysis A statistical technique that provides information about the dependent variable for each level of independent variable after adjustment for covariation. It is a more versatile variation of multiple regression analysis and analysis of covariance.

multiple comparison procedures Statistical tests applied after an ANOVA when there is a difference between groups to determine which pairs of means are different from one another. Also called a post hoc test.

multiple correlation coefficient (R) A statistic that summarizes the degree and direction of the relationship between two or more independent variables, grouped together, and a dependent variable.

multiple regression A statistical method for calculating the equation that describes the direction and strength of the relationship between two or more independent variables and one dependent variable.

multiplicity problem A situation that occurs when a large number of statistical tests are conducted on the same data. There is a tendency to reject some of the null hypotheses even when all of the null hypotheses are true.

multistage sampling A sampling method that occurs in stages from larger units to smaller units.

multitrait-multimethod approach A method to establish the construct validity of an instrument, which assesses convergence and divergence among different tests of the phenomenon with the same group of subjects. The approach involves comparison of the scores obtained with a test that measures the construct and a test that measures a different construct (such as the opposite construct) and comparison of the results of two different tests of the same construct.

multivariate analysis of variance (MANOVA) A multivariate statistical technique similar to ANOVA used when there is more than one dependent variable. This technique is used to test simultaneously the means of two or more groups on two or more dependent variables.

multivariate analysis of covariance (MANCOVA) A multivariate statistical technique similar to ANCOVA used when there are covariates and more than one dependent variable.

multivariate approach Research designs to study multiple independent or dependent variables.

multivariate statistics Statistical procedures used to analyze the relationships among three or more variables simultaneously.

mutually exclusive categories Categories set up so that no observation can be classified into more than one category.

N The total number of subjects in the sample.

n The number of subjects in a subgroup of the sample.

narrow-range theory A theory with limited generalizability with a focus on one phenomenon at one point in time.

naturalistic inquiry A design in which observations obtained in the natural setting are used to answer the research question.

naturalistic paradigm A perspective of the world in which truth is seen as dynamic and seen in real historical, social, and cultural contexts.

naturalistic setting A setting in which the subjects are commonly found, whether or not they are in a research study.

needs assessment A systematic collection of data to determine the needs of a group or agency to set policy or allocate resources.

negative case analysis A process in qualitative research to determine credibility of findings through analysis of observations that differ from expected findings.

negative correlation See negative relationship.

negative relationship A negative correlation between two variables, such that an increase in one variable is associated with a decrease in the other variable. Also called negative correlation or inverse relationship.

negative results Research results that do not support the research hypothesis or theoretical framework for the study and accept the null hypothesis.

negatively skewed distribution A graphic display in which the distribution of values contains a large number of high values, resulting in a longer tail on the left of the distribution curve.

negativity bias An effect in which the participant responds negatively to each question.

network sampling See snowball sampling.

nominal data/measure The lowest level of data measurement with data assigned to mutually exclusive categories with arbitrary number labels.

nominal scale A level of measurement for categorical variables. All observations with the same characteristic are placed in a category (named) and are considered equivalent. A nominal scale is the least complex scale of measurement.

nondirectional hypothesis A hypothesis that does not specify the direction of the difference between the independent and dependent variables. The sampling distribution curve is divided into two equal parts at each end of the distribution to determine the values needed to reject the null hypothesis. Also called a two-tailed hypothesis.

nonequivalent control group A control comparison group that is not composed of randomly assigned individuals; therefore, it may be different (not equivalent) than the experimental group prior to the experimental treatment.

nonequivalent control group design A quasi-experimental design in which there are pretest/post-test observations and nonrandom assignment of subjects into experimental and control groups.

nonexperimental research A research study in which the researcher collects data without conducting any intervention or experimental treatment.

nonmonotonic relationship Correlation in which there is a change in direction and degree of association between X and Y over the distribution of values.

nonparametric statistics Inferential statistical tests that require less restrictive distribution assumptions than parametric statistics; statistical tests often used with nominal or ordinal data or with small sample sizes. Also called distribution-free statistics.

nonparticipant observer—covert The researcher or observer who does not interact with subjects, remains unidentified, and does not provide information about the study to the subjects.

nonparticipant observer—overt The researcher who does not interact with subjects but is identified and provides information about data collection to the subjects.

nonprobability sample A sample consisting of participants assigned by nonrandom methods as a convenience or to achieve a purpose or quota.

nonpuriousness An assurance that variables other than the independent variable have been ruled out in determination of the cause of the effect on the dependent variable.

nonrefereed journal A journal that uses editorial staff or consultants rather than an expert peer review panel to review manuscripts for publication.

nonschedule interview A standardized interview in which the researcher is free to vary the order and phrasing of questions.

nonsignificant result (NS) The result of a statistical test that indicates that the findings could be due to chance rather than to other causes, according to the predetermined level of significance set by the researcher.

nonsymmetrical distribution A continuous frequency distribution of values in which there is a high frequency of high or low values (skewed distribution) across the distribution; the distribution is off center.

normal curve See normal distribution.

normal distribution A continuous frequency distribution of values with a symmetrical, unimodal, bell-shaped curve in which half of the values are above the mean and the other half below the mean. Also called a normal curve or Gaussian curve.

norms Standards for test performance used for comparison of individual or group scores. The standards are based on results from testing of large samples.

normative theory Theory developed to describe, explain, or predict values based on consistency and logic of underlying assumptions, rather than empirical testing.

norm-referenced measurement Technique in which the scores for an individual are compared with a standardized norm or the values obtained in the rest of the sample.

null hypothesis (H$_0$) A statistical hypothesis that states that there is no difference between the population means and that any difference is due to chance. Also called the statistical hypothesis.

nursing research The systematic, objective study of phenomena of interest to the discipline of nursing using naturalistic or scientific methods.

nursing science The body of knowledge specific to nursing that guides nursing practice and research.

objectivity The process of remaining without judgment and bias in the conduct of scientific research to the extent that another independent researcher would obtain similar results concurrently.

oblique factor rotation In factor analysis, a statistical technique to produce correlated factors during which the rotating axes depart from a 90-degree angle.

observation Collection of data through visual observation of people experiencing the phenomenon.

observational notes See field notes.

observational research A research study to answer questions about phenomena in which data are collected through visual observation of the people experiencing the phenomena.

observed score The actual score or numeric value assigned to or achieved by an individual on a measure, which includes the true score and error. Also called the obtained score.

obtained score See observed score.

one-group pretest/post-test design A pre-experimental research design in which observations are made on a group of subjects before and after an experimental treatment to measure the effect of the treatment.

one-shot case study A pre-experimental research design in which observations are made on a group of subjects who have received a treatment to measure the effects of the treatment. No pretreatment observations are conducted.

one-way analysis of variance An analysis of variance test to measure the relationship between one independent variable and a dependent variable.

one-tailed hypothesis See directional hypothesis.

one-tailed test A test of statistical significance used with a directional hypothesis in which the values critical to determine statistical significance occur in only one tail, the right or the left, of the sampling distribution.

ontology A study of the nature of reality.

open coding The first level in data analysis in grounded theory, which involves examining, comparing, conceptualizing, and categorizing data from narrative records.

open-ended question Questions that allow the participants to respond with their own unrestricted words and ideas instead of choosing from a fixed set of responses.

operational definition The definition of a construct or variable that describes how it will be measured or observed. Also known as epistemic definitions, rules of correspondence, or rules of interpretation.

operationalization The process of describing how concepts will be observed or measured.

ordinal data/measure The second level of data measurement in which data are categorized into mutually exclusive and exhaustive categories and ranked in order of magnitude along some attribute or dimension. The differences between levels of magnitude are not equal.

ordinal scale A level of measurement in which numbers are used to indicate the rank order of magnitude of observations along a dimension, such as class rank, but they do not indicate the magnitude of difference. This scale is more complex than a nominal scale and less complex than an interval scale.

ordinary least squares (OLS) See least-squares estimation.

ordinate See Y-axis.

orthogonal factor rotation In factor analysis, a factor rotation procedure in which factors are kept independent, or at 90-degree angles to one another, so that factors are uncorrelated with one another.

outcome analysis See impact analysis.

outcome variable A term that refers to the dependent variable; a measure of the outcome or the effect in a study.

outliers Extreme numerical values or codes that lie outside the coding scheme and are remote from one another on a graphic display of the distribution.

***p* value** In statistical testing, the probability that the results obtained are due to chance; the probability of a type 1 error.

pair-matching See matching.

pairwise deletion A process to delete cases with missing data on a selective basis.

panel design See panel study.

panel of experts See expert panel.

panel study A type of longitudinal study in which data are collected from two or more cohorts at two or more data collection times. The design allows observation of similarities and differences in cohorts and change over time. Also called a panel design.

paradigm A way of looking at the world or a perspective on phenomena that presents a set of interrelated philosophical assumptions about the world. The perspective guides research and practice.

parallel form reliability See alternate form reliability.

parameter A numerical characteristic of a population, such as the average family income, for a specified group.

parametric statistics Inferential statistical tests that require specific distributional assumptions for the variable. The level of data measurement is interval or ratio, the values are normally distributed, and the values have equal variation in the population.

participant An individual who provides information in a research study. Also called the study participant.

participant observation A method of data collection in which the researcher collects information about a group as an interactive member of the group.

participant observer—covert The researcher or observer who interacts with the subjects and collects information without informing them about the research.

participant observer—overt The researcher or observer who interacts with the subjects and collects information after informing them about the research.

path analysis A statistical testing procedure based on multiple regression techniques used to test a causal model in an attempt to explain the causes of phenomena, typically using nonexperimental data. The researcher hypothesizes the relationships and order of relationships among variables and then tests the strength of the relationships.

path coefficient The weight representing the effect of one variable on another in path analysis.

path diagram A graphic display of the hypothesized relationships and causal flow among variables in a causal model.

patiency In prescriptive theory, the recipients of prescriptions.

pattern The shape, repetition, and variation of an event or phenomenon.

Pearson's *r* A commonly used correlation coefficient to describe the magnitude and direction of an association between two variables measured at least at the interval level of data measurement. Also called the Pearson's product-moment correlation.

Pearson's product-moment correlation See Pearson's *r*.

peer-reviewed journal See refereed journal.

percentage (%) A statistic that refers to the proportion of a subset to the total set or group, expressed as a percent ranging from 0 to 100.

percentile A measure of rank; the percentage of cases below a given score.

peer review The process in which manuscripts, research reports, or research proposals are reviewed and critiqued by other experts or researchers in the field for the purpose of making recommendations for publication or funding.

peer reviewer A person with content or research expertise or experience who participates in the peer review process.

perfect correlation/relationship An association or relationship in which the values of one variable exactly predict the values of another variable, expressed as +1.00 or −1.00.

personal notes In field studies, written notes taken during a study to record the observer's personal feelings or thoughts.

personal interview A direct face-to-face or telephone interview between a researcher and a participant.

personality inventories Self-report measures used to determine differences in personality traits, values, needs, or other attributes in participants.

phenomena See phenomenon.

phenomenological method A qualitative research approach based on constructing and describing the meaning of an experience through intensive discussion with people living the experience.

phenomenological reduction A term that refers to recovery of original awareness of a phenomenon.

phenomenological research Research conducted using phenomenological methods to describe an experience as it is lived.

phenomenology A perspective originating from philosophy and psychology that focuses on understanding subjects' lived experience of some phenomenon and their interpretation of that experience.

phenomenon The abstract idea, concept, observation, event, or variable under study; plural is phenomena.

phi coefficient A statistical indicator describing the magnitude of the relationship between two dichotomous variables.

philosophical research Research based on the study of reality, truth, and the principles of existence, knowledge, and conduct.

physiological measurement The use of instruments to obtain physical and biological measurements.

pie charts A graphic description of the frequency distribution depicted as proportions (slices) of a circle (pie).

pilot To conduct a pilot study.

pilot study/project A trial run with a small-scale study prior to conducting a major study to provide an opportunity to test and refine procedures or to obtain preliminary information.

pink sheet The evaluation form containing the comments and priority score assigned by the peer review panel for a grant proposal submitted to the National Institutes of Health.

platykurtotic distribution A distribution with a flattened peak.

plethysmography Procedure to measure changes in volume.

point estimation A procedure in which the researcher makes statistical inferences about a population parameter based on the results obtained in a sample.

policy research Research conducted to obtain information needed to create and implement policy.

population The entire set of individuals or objects that have a common characteristic or set of criteria, such as college freshmen.

population mean The estimated mean for the entire population based on the sample means.

population validity The ability to generalize the results to other populations.

positive correlation See positive relationship.

positively skewed distribution A graphic display in which the distribution of values contains a large number of high values, resulting in a longer tail on the right of the distribution curve.

positive relationship A positive correlation between two variables, such that an increase in one variable is associated with an increase in the other variable, or a decrease in one corresponds with a decrease in the other. Also called a positive correlation.

positive results Research results that support the research hypothesis or theoretical framework for the study; a rejection of the null hypothesis.

positivist-empiricist paradigm See positivist paradigm.

positivist paradigm The traditional scientific objective view of the world, which assumes that reality can be objectively measured and observed, independent of historical, social, or cultural contexts. This perspective forms the basis for quantitative experimental research oriented toward development of universal principles and outcomes. Also called the positivist-empiricist paradigm.

post hoc tests Additional tests conducted after a statistical procedure. See multiple comparison methods.

post-test Collection of data after the implementation of an experimental treatment.

post-test only design See post-test only control group design.

post-test only control group design An experimental design in which data are collected from subjects only after the implementation of the experimental treatment. Also called an after only design or post-test only design.

postulate A statement to describe an assumed relationship between concepts.

power The ability of a research design to detect relationships among variables in a study; the probability of correctly rejecting a false null hypothesis.

power analysis A statistical procedure (1) for determining the required sample size, also called the Cohen power test, (2) for estimating the likelihood of committing a type II error.

power of a statistical test The ability of a test to detect small, statistically significant differences or relationships to reject the null hypothesis when it should be rejected.

practice theory Theory that can be validated at the practice level.

precision The quality of being explicit, clear, and able to differentiate from similar concepts, attributes, or measurement values.

predictability See stability.

prediction The use of empirical evidence to determine the relationship among variables in a different setting or sample at some time in the future; description of the variables that will result in the desired outcome.

prediction study A nonexperimental research design in which a researcher makes forecasts for the future based on selected phenomena.

predictive theory A theory composed of interrelated concepts and propositional statements that forecast an outcome.

predictive validity A criterion of validity of an instrument that refers to the ability of the instrument to predict behavior of subjects in the future; the degree of correlation between current and future measurements of a concept.

predictor variable See independent variable.

preexisting data Information collected for purposes other than the current research study.

pre-experimental design A type of experimental research design in which the researcher has minimal control over the study, such as a one-shot case study and the one-group pretest/post-test design.

prescriptive theory A theory that intends to control or change phenomena by specifying actions and interventions that will facilitate achievement of a goal.

present-mindedness An analysis of data collected at an earlier time period from a current perspective.

pretest An instrument to collect data or observations from subjects before the introduction of an experimental intervention.

pretest/post-test design An experimental design in which data are collected from subjects before and after the introduction of an experimental intervention. Also called a before–after design.

pretest/post-test control group design True experimental design in which subjects are randomly assigned to the control and experimental groups, and data are collected from both groups before and after an experimental treatment.

prevalence The number of cases of a disease or other condition in a specified population at a particular point or period of time.

prevalence study A study to determine the number of existing cases at or during a specified period of time.

primary analysis The initial analysis of data.

primary source The original firsthand report or first research report of an event, experience, or research findings. Examples of firsthand reports include archival materials, private journals, public or private letters, films, tapes, artifacts, and records, which may or may not contain critical analyses.

principal axis factoring In factor analysis, the procedure to analyze common factor variance, using estimates of the communality on the diagonal of the correlation matrix.

principal components analysis In factor analysis, the procedure to extract factors by maximizing the amount of variance and extracting the first factor, then applying the same method to extract the second factor and each other factor.

principal investigator The primary researcher in a study or the researcher funded and responsible for the development and implementation of a study.

principle of discontinuity In factor analysis, a procedure in which the percentage of variance explained by each factor is graphed. Factors that occur after the point at which there is a drop in the percentage of variance explained are dropped. Also called the scree test.

print data bases Print indexes, such as card catalogs, indexes, and abstract reviews, used to locate research reports and conceptual articles in journals and professional or government publications.

privacy The ethical right to minimal intrusion, including protecting anonymity and confidentiality of subjects.

probability The relative frequency or likelihood of an event in repeated trials under similar test conditions.

probability level (p) See level of significance.

probability sample A sample selected through random sampling procedures.

probability sampling The process of selecting a sample from the population through random sampling procedures. Examples of types of probability sampling include simple, stratified, cluster, and systematic random sampling techniques.

probe A prompt, phrase, or question used by an interviewer to encourage an additional response or elaboration on a point or discussion topic.

problem statement A focused question or statement that provides information about the problem to be solved and what type of answer or information is needed.

process analysis An evaluation of the method through which an intervention or program is implemented in practice.

process consent The continuous, transactional negotiation with subjects regarding ongoing participation in qualitative research.

process evaluation See formative evaluation research.

product-moment correlation (*r*) See Pearson's *r*.

product testing A type of research to test medical devices or other products in the clinical setting.

program evaluation A formative or summative evaluation of the implementation or outcome of a project or program.

projective technique A self-report measure in which the investigator asks the subject to respond to ambiguous, unstructured, external stimuli. The response reflects the respondent's feelings projected on the stimuli.

prolonged engagement In qualitative research, the process of taking time to develop an in-depth understanding of the group and phenomena under study to achieve data credibility.

proportion A type of ratio in which the value for the numerator is included in the denominator, and the resultant value is stated as a percentage.

proportional stratified sampling A random sampling technique in which subjects are selected from layers (strata) in the population in proportion to the size of the layer in the total population.

proportionate sample A research sample selected through proportionate stratified sampling procedures.

proportionate sampling design A study plan in which data are obtained from a proportionate sample.

proposal A written document detailing what the researcher plans or proposes to study. The proposal includes the research problem, its significance, methods and procedures for data collection and analysis, and the fiscal budget if the proposal seeks funding. Also called the research proposal.

proposition A statement about the relationship among concepts that lays the foundation for development of theory and methods for testing relationships.

prospective design See prospective study.

prospective study Study in which an independent variable is identified at the present time, and the subjects are followed up on to observe the effect on the dependent variable in the future. Also called cohort study.

protocol The formal guidelines and procedures for the implementation of a study. Also called study protocol.

proxy measure A substitute measure of a variable that cannot be directly measured.

psychometric assessment An evaluation of the quality of an instrument based on evidence of validity and reliability. Also called psychometric evaluation.

psychometric evaluation See psychometric assessment.

psychometric properties The technical qualities of an instrument, especially the validity and reliability, and the procedures used in developing and testing the instrument.

psychometrics The theory and development of measurement instruments and techniques.

public funding agencies Tax-supported government agencies that supply financial support for research or other projects.

pure research See basic research.

purpose The goal or intent of the research study. Also called the aim, study aim, statement of purpose, or study purpose.

purposive sample Nonprobability sampling in which the researcher selects subjects who are most typical and likely to represent the phenomenon of research interest. Also called a judgmental sample.

Q methodology See Q-sort.

Q-sort A data collection procedure to determine the subject's degree of agreement or disagreement with an idea in which subjects sort statements into categories consistent with their attitudes or ratings of the statements.

qualitative analysis The systematic summation and interpretation of non-numeric data to reveal the meaning and pattern of relationships.

qualitative data Narrative information collected in a qualitative study.

qualitative measurement The assignment of items or observations to mutually exclusive categories that represent the variation in the concepts under observation.

qualitative research Descriptive study to collect and analyze in-depth narrative data that provide information about the subjective meaning of human experiences and phenomena, usually conducted in the natural setting. Also called qualitative study.

qualitative study See qualitative research.

quantitative analysis The systematic statistical manipulation and analysis of numerical data to describe phenomena or the numerical relationships among them.

quantitative data Numeric data collected in a quantitative study.

quantitative measurement The assignment of numbers from one set to another set of items, events, or behaviors based on a rule; the sets or numerical categories represent the value or amount of a characteristic.

quantitative research Research study that collects numerical data and is based on objectivity, measurement, control of the situation, and the ability to generalize findings.

quartimax In factor analysis, a method to simplify variables by increasing the dispersion of the loadings within the variables across factors.

quasi-experiment A study using a quasi-experimental design.

quasi-experimental design A research design in which there is manipulation of the independent variable and measures to control, but there is nonrandom assignment of subjects into treatment and control groups or no control group.

quasi-statistics In qualitative analysis, using numbers in the analysis of qualitative data, such as counting and comparing patterns and frequencies.

query letter A letter sent to an editor of a journal to inquire if the editor is interested in publication of a manuscript. The letter usually includes a statement about why the content is important and an outline of the contents of the manuscript.

questionnaire Self-administered paper and pencil instrument developed to obtain information from participants in a research study. Also called a self-administered questionnaire.

quota sample A sample obtained through quota sampling techniques.

quota sampling A nonprobability sampling technique in which the subjects are selected in proportions representative of the same strata in the population.

R

r See Pearson's *r*.

R See multiple correlation coefficient.

R^2 See squared multiple correlation coefficient.

random assignment A procedure used in an experimental study to ensure that each subject has an equal chance of being assigned to any one of the treatment or control groups.

random digit dialing A variation of cluster sampling in which all the telephone numbers in an area comprise the population for sampling.

random error Measurement errors that are unpredictable and highly variable.

randomization list In a clinical trial, the list of random assignments kept by a person other than the researcher who treats subjects or evaluates their responses.

randomization test A nonparametric test used with small samples having multiple applications of conditions over time to determine differences in data in each of the conditions.

randomized block design A method to control potentially extraneous variables by including them as independent variables and randomly assigning individuals with and without the characteristic to separate treatment groups. For example, to control for gender, men would be randomly assigned to men's treatment and control groups and women would be randomly assigned to women's treatment and control groups, with the results for all four groups compared.

random number table A table of hundreds of numbers constructed in such a way that each number 0 through 9 has a probability of one in ten chances of occurring in any position in the table, and the occurrence of any number in any position is independent of the occurrence of any number in any other position in the table. The table is used for randomization procedures. Also called table of random numbers.

random sample A sample obtained by chance through random assignment procedures.

randomization The random assignment of subjects to treatment groups.

range (1) A measure of variation in scores; the distance between the minimum and maximum values in a set of values or scores computed by subtracting the minimum score from the maximum score. (2) In an instrument, the measure includes all variations in intensity, amplitude, and frequency.

rate A form of proportion that includes specification of the point or period of time.

rating scale An instrument that asks the subject to select the most closely representative response from a range of possible responses or values.

ratio data Data that have the properties of rank order and equal intervals relative to an absolute zero, such as height and weight.

ratio level of measurement The highest form of measurement in which there is rank order and equal magnitude of difference for intervals relative to an absolute zero.

ratio scale A scale in which there is rank order and equal magnitude of difference between points on the scale along a dimension with an absolute zero. Examples are scales for height and weight.

raw data Data in the form in which they were originally collected with no additional manipulation or coding.

reactivity A threat to the external validity of a study in which the subjects change their responses because they know they are being observed, which may bias the results of the study.

reactive effects of the pretest A threat to the external validity of a study in which the subject's response to the pretest changes the subject's response to treatment and later measurement.

readability The degree of difficulty in reading and understanding the words used in research instruments by people with varied reading skills. Readability can be evaluated with readability formulas.

real duration The actual length of time over which an event or phenomenon occurred.

real frequency The actual number of times an event or phenomenon occurred in a specified time period.

recommendation Application of a study to practice, education, development of theory, or future research.

rectangular matrix A variable by subject matrix of data with no missing entries.

recursive model A path model with unidirectional causation and no feedback loops.

references   The list of books, articles, or other sources of information cited in a manuscript or research report.

refereed journal   A journal that uses peer experts to review manuscripts for recommendation for publication. Also called peer-reviewed journal.

reflexive   In qualitative research, a term that refers to the dual source of insight from being both researcher and participant.

reflexive critique   A qualitative research data analysis technique in which the researcher and participants engage in dialogue to reveal each person's interpretation of the meaning of the experience.

region of rejection   See critical region.

regression   A statistical procedure for calculating the equation that describes the linear relationship between one or more independent variables and a dependent variable.

regression coefficient   The regression intercept and slope in bivariate regression. In multiple regression, the numbers that represent the regression equation.

relationship   The connection or association between two or more variables.

relative frequency   The ratio of the frequency observed for a category divided by the total number of observations for all categories in the data set.

reliability   The proportion of true variance to total variance; the consistency and dependability of an instrument to measure a variable. The types of reliability are stability, equivalence, and internal consistency reliability.

reliability coefficient   A term that refers to the degree of reliability of an instrument expressed as a value ranging from 0.0 to 1.0; the relationship between true variance, error variance, and total variance. Statistical techniques to establish reliability are the Cronbach's alpha, split-half, test–retest, and inter-rater reliability approaches.

repeated measures design An experimental design in which subjects receive more than one experimental treatment or condition in random order. A type of crossover design.

replication The process of repeating or duplicating a study.

replication study A research study that repeats or duplicates a study following the same design and procedures to determine whether the findings can be repeated, usually with a different sample or setting.

representativeness The degree to which the key characteristics of the sample or other subset resembles the larger characteristics of the total population.

representative sample A sample with key characteristics similar to the characteristics of the population.

reproducibility The ability of an instrument to give equal output in response to equal input or the ability to which a process can be reproduced under variable circumstances.

research The systematic, logical inquiry into the nature of phenomena to develop knowledge.

research abstract See abstract.

research base The accumulated body of knowledge accrued from a number of research studies about the phenomena.

research control See control.

research design The general plan for the methods and procedures of a study.

research ethics See ethics.

research hypothesis (H₁) A hypothesis that states the researcher's expectations about the outcomes of the study, the alternative to the statistical null hypothesis. Also called the scientific, substantive, or theoretical hypothesis.

research instruments See instruments.

research literature See data-based literature.

research methods See methods.

research problem A situation or question that is amenable to investigation. A statement that presents the question to be answered in the research study.

research proposal See proposal.

research question A statement of the question or inquiry to be answered in the research investigation into a research problem.

research report A written or oral summary of the question, methods, findings, and implications of a research study.

research tools See instruments.

research topic The concept, event, behavior, condition, or other phenomenon of interest in a research study.

research utilization The systematic method of implementation and evaluation of research-based interventions in practice or application in a situation unrelated to the original intention of the original study. Also called utilization.

residuals In multiple regression statistics, the unexplained variance or the error term; the difference between the actual values of the dependent variable and the estimated values of the dependent variable determined by the regression equation.

respect for people The ethical perspective that people have the right to self-determination and to being treated as autonomous individuals, including the freedom to partici-pate or not participate in research.

respondent The individual who responds or answers questions presented by the researcher.

response rate The ratio of the number of people who participate in a research study compared with the number of people invited to participate.

response-set bias The error of measurement due to the tendency of a participant to respond in a characteristic way regardless of the content of the question, such as consistently high or in agreement with each question.

results The findings or answers to research questions or hypotheses obtained through systematic collection and analysis of data.

retrospective design A research plan to conduct retro-spective research.

retrospective research A research study in which the dependent variable (the effect) is identified in the present, and the researcher investigates variables that occurred in the past to determine possible independent variables (the causes). The design may include a comparison group of people similar in other aspects except for the absence of the dependent variable.

revelatory case A case that provides a researcher with the opportunity to investigate a phenomenon previously unavailable to research.

review of available data A study conducted on existing data, including data not specifically collected for research purposes.

review of literature A systematic, critical study of the most significant published scholarly literature on a topic.

R_n **test of ranks** A nonparametric test to evaluate differences in ranking of behavior change among the various baselines used with small samples with multiple baselines.

rights of subjects The ethical considerations for human subjects involved in research, including the protection from harm, protection of vulnerable subjects, right to be informed, right to participate voluntarily, and right to protection of privacy.

risks Potential negative or harmful effects from participation in a study.

risk/benefit ratio The proportion in which risk or harm to human subjects is minimized and benefits of the study are maximized; the relative costs and benefits of a study to the subject and to society.

rival hypothesis An alternative explanation for understanding the results of a study, which is in disagreement with the research hypothesis.

robust A statistic that remains useful even with the violation of underlying assumptions.

rotated factor matrix The product of the second phase of factor analysis, in which the factors have been manipulated to show how every variable is correlated with the factor to allow the researcher to interpret the patterns and themes for each factor.

rows The horizontal data in a table.

rules of correspondence See operational definition.

rules of interpretation See operational definition.

S

sample A subset *(n)* of the entire population *(N)*, selected for a study to represent the entire population.

sampling The process of selecting a group or sample of subjects from the entire population for participation in a research study.

sampling bias (1) A threat to the external validity of a study that occurs when random sampling procedures are not used. (2) Differences between sample data and population data attributable to sampling procedures.

sampling distribution A theoretical distribution that would occur using an infinite number of random samples from the population.

sampling error Random fluctuations in data that occur in different samples from the same population.

sampling frame A listing of all the elements in the population from which the sample is selected.

sampling unit The unit used for sample selection.

SAQ Self-administered questionnaire. See questionnaire.

saturation In grounded theory research, the situation in which there is repetition and redundancy in the data collected, at which point the data collection is considered complete.

scale A measure of an attribute consisting of a series of related items to which the subject responds. The subject's score on the measure represents a point along a continuum that represents a dimension of the attribute.

scaling The assignment of a composite score to an attribute based on a combination of several measurements.

scalogram analysis Procedure to examine whether a cumulative scale is unidimensional and reproducible, in which the total score reflects the score on the items.

scatter diagram See scatter plot.

scattergram See scatter plot.

scatter plot A graphic picture of the relationship between two variables in which dots represent the point of intersection for pairs of X and Y variables. Also called scatter diagram or scattergram.

schedule The list of questions that make up a questionnaire or interview guide.

Scheffé's test A post hoc test used to test differences in all possible pairs of means; used after a significant ANOVA.

schematic model A conceptual model that portrays a phenomenon with a figurative display of the relationships among concepts comprising the phenomenon.

scholarly literature See data-based literature.

scientific hypothesis See research hypothesis.

scientific method An orderly, systematic, controlled approach to obtaining precise empirical information and testing ideas.

scientific observation Data collection based on systematic, objective, and controlled planning, collecting, and recording of information relevant to scientific concepts and theories.

scientific merit The degree to which a study is methodologically and conceptually sound, theoretically relevant, and internally and externally valid.

scientific theory Testable theory that describes, explains, and predicts the empirical world.

scree test See principle of discontinuity.

screening instrument An instrument used to determine whether or not subjects meet the eligibility criteria for a study.

seasonal variability Fluctuation that occurs in a pattern corresponding with changes in seasons.

secondary analysis A form of research in which a set of existing data is analyzed by another researcher to test the same or a new research hypothesis, or analyzed by the same researcher to test a new research hypothesis.

secondary source (1) In the research literature, a report or synopsis of a research study by someone other than the researchers. (2) In historical research, materials such as newspaper or journal articles from the period of time being studied that cite secondhand opinions and interpretations of an event by someone who did not directly experience an event.

selection bias A threat to the internal validity of an experimental study that occurs when pretreatment differences between groups (such as self-selected groups) may account for the differences in results, rather than the treatment condition.

selective sampling In grounded theory, the process of selecting relevant data from the data set.

self-administered questionnaire (SAQ) See questionnaire.

self-determination A person's right to a voluntary decision whether to participate in a research study.

self-report A data collection procedure in which the subject directly provides information, frequently by interview or questionnaire.

self-selection A sample selection procedure in which subjects volunteer to participate in a study.

semantic differential An attitude scale that asks respondents to select a point that corresponds to their attitude on a seven-point rating scale. The points are anchored by two descriptive words or phrases representing bipolar attitudes about a concept.

semiquartile range The portion of values obtained by dividing the values in the middle half (50%) of a frequency distribution in half.

semistructured interview An interview in which the interviewer asks specified questions and uses discretionary probes or asks additional questions to amplify and clarify responses.

sensitivity In measurement, the degree to which an instrument is able to discriminate among different amounts of the variable being measured.

sentence completion technique A descriptive instrument in which the respondent is asked to finish an incomplete sentence. A useful technique for assessment of feelings and attitudes.

sequence effects Effects based on the sequencing of treatments or events, rather than the treatment itself.

sequential comparison design The use of a subject's baseline as a control comparison for values obtained after the treatment condition.

serendipitous findings Unanticipated research results.

setting A description of the physical location and conditions under which data were collected.

significance level The probability that a relationship could be caused by chance or error. A significance level of .01 means that the relationship would be found by chance only one time out of 100.

sign system In structured observation research, the listing of behaviors that may occur prior to conducting the study and used to record behaviors observed during the study.

sign test A nonparametric statistical test that is used to test hypotheses about population medians or differences in population medians.

signed rank A rank given the sign of the corresponding observation.

simple hypothesis A hypothesis that predicts the relationship between the independent variable and the dependent variable.

simple random sampling A sampling procedure using random selection methods to ensure each unit in the population has an equal and independent chance of being selected.

simulation studies A study to observe participant behavior or responses to laboratory situations or case studies developed to represent reality.

single-blind study A research study in which either the researcher does not know which subjects are in the experimental group or the control group but the subjects know to which group they belong, or the subjects do not know whether they are in the experimental group or the control group, but the researcher knows which subjects are in each group.

situated In qualitative research, the term that identifies the position of the researcher within the group under study.

skewed distribution An asymmetrical frequency distribution of values with a peak at one end of the distribution and a long tail at the opposite end.

slope The steepness rate at which a horizontal line rises across a table of values.

snowball sampling A sampling procedure in which subjects are located based on referrals from other subjects in the sample. Also called network sampling.

social desirability response set A bias in self-reporting that occurs when subjects have a tendency to respond in a manner most socially acceptable or pleasing to the researcher rather than revealing their true attitudes or opinions.

social history The study of society at a period in time to understand the values and beliefs in routine daily life during that time.

social situation In qualitative research, a term that refers to the activities of the actors, the members of the cultural group under study, in a designated place.

Solomon four-group design A true experimental design that uses a pretest/post-test design for one pair of experimental and control groups and a post-test only design for a second pair of experimental and control groups to minimize threats to internal and external validity.

Spearman-Brown prophecy formula An equation for correcting a reliability estimate that was calculated by the split-half method.

Spearman rank-order correlation coefficient A nonparametric measure of the degree of magnitude and direction of the relationship between two variables measured on the ordinal (rank order) scale or when one or both variables is skewed or has an outlier. Also called Spearman's rho.

Spearman's rho See Spearman's rank-order correlation coefficient.

specificity The ability of an instrument to measure only the phenomenon of interest and ignore extraneous or competing phenomena.

split-half reliability See split-half technique.

split-half technique A procedure for measuring the internal consistency reliability of an instrument in which the scores on half of the measure are correlated with scores on the other half. Also called split-half reliability.

spread of a distribution The variability, amount of distance, and width between the high and low values of a distribution.

SPSS A trademark name for a statistical software package for the social sciences.

spurious associations A relationship between two variables based on the influence of a third variable.

squared multiple correlation coefficient (R^2) A statistic from multiple regression that indicates the proportion of variance in the dependent variable explained by a group of independent variables.

stability reliability The degree of consistency (predictability) of a research instrument over time as evidenced by test–retest procedures on repeated measures with the instrument. Also called dependability.

standard deviation (SD, s) A statistical measure of variability that indicates the average variation from the mean value for all values in the data set; the square root of the variance.

standard error The standard deviation of the sampling distribution, usually the distribution of the mean.

standard error of estimate The standard deviation of the errors from the regression line in regression analysis used to estimate the accuracy of the regression predictions.

standardized interview An interview following a set format.

standard scores Scores expressed in terms of standard deviations from the mean, with the scores transformed to have a mean of 0 and standard deviation of 1.0.

statement of purpose See purpose.

statistic A numerical index of a sample that is used to estimate the population parameter.

statistical analysis The organization and analysis of numerical data using descriptive and inferential statistical procedures.

statistical control A statistical technique to control or isolate the effect of extraneous variance on the dependent variable.

statistical hypothesis See null hypothesis.

statistical inference The process of making conclusions about the population based on results obtained with a sample.

statistical model The mathematical equations that express the direction and magnitude of relationships among the variables.

statistical power analysis A statistical technique for estimating the effectiveness of a test in rejecting false null hypotheses.

statistical regression The tendency of extreme scores, which are unstable, to change in the direction of the mean.

statistical reliability A measure of the internal consistency of responses to all items at one time on a form of a measure.

statistical significance A term that indicates that the results obtained in the analysis of the data from the sample are unlikely to be due to chance according to the preset level of probability.

statistical test A procedure in which the researcher determines the probability that the results of the analysis of the data from the sample reflect the results of the population.

stem question The attitude or phenomenon to be rated on a scale.

stepwise multiple regression analysis A statistical procedure for analyzing the simultaneous effect of multiple variables on the dependent variable. The independent variable that is most highly correlated with the dependent variable is entered into the regression equation first, followed by the second most highly correlated independent variable, then the third and other variables until all the variables have been entered into the equation. Also called forward stepwise multiple regression analysis. Other techniques in stepwise regression include the backward and stepwise solutions, and maximum R^2 improvement technique.

stipend A financial award to research subjects to serve as an incentive for participation or to compensate for expenses.

strata Subgroups of the population divided according to certain characteristics important to the study.

stratified random sample A random sample obtained by stratified sampling procedures.

stratified sampling A procedure in which a random sample is selected in proportion to each independent stratum or subgroup in the population. The subgroups represent characteristics important to the study.

structured data collection A method of data collection in which the response categories are determined by the researcher prior to the data collection.

structured interviews Interviews in which the interviewer uses the same procedure and set of questions with every participant.

structured observational technique A research situation in which the researcher sets criteria for what is to be observed prior to the observation and follows the criteria using a checklist or schedule to record the observations.

study aim See purpose.

study participant See participant.

study protocol See protocol.

study purpose See purpose.

study section The initial peer group that reviews grant applications to the National Institutes of Health.

student's *t*-test See *t*-test.

subgroup effects The different effects of the independent variable on the dependent variable within subsets of the sample.

subjects The participants who provide data in a research study.

substantive hypothesis See research hypothesis.

summated rating scale See Likert scale.

summative evaluation research Research conducted at the conclusion of a program or intervention to evaluate the quality or effectiveness of the program.

survey A self-report instrument used to gather information on the characteristics of a population or to obtain information on a topic.

survey research A type of nonexperimental study in which the researcher gathers self-report data from a sample to determine the characteristics of a population or obtain information on a topic.

survival analysis See life table analysis.

symbolic interactionism A philosophical belief system based on the assumption that humans learn about and define the world through social interactions and symbolic communication.

symmetric distribution A frequency distribution in which both halves of the distribution are the same.

systematic error   The error attributed to characteristics of the subject that do not fluctuate or change over time, or to improper calibration of an instrument.

systematic random sampling   A random sampling procedure in which members of the population or sampling frame are selected for the study at fixed intervals, such as the selection of every 10th individual.

systematic replication   Repeated replication of a study with systematic alteration of conditions to determine which factors in the experiment produce similar results.

t **distribution**   A symmetrical distribution that resembles a normal distribution.

t-**test (***t***)**   A parametric statistical test to analyze the difference between means of two groups of values to determine whether they are different by chance or another factor. The values must be obtained at the interval or ratio level of measurement. If the samples are not independent (related), a paired or correlated *t*-test would be used. Also called the student's *t*-test.

table of random numbers   See random number table.

tables   Summaries of statistical information to display results in a research report.

table shells   A table without numbers prepared as a guide for data analysis.

tacit knowledge   Information commonly known by members of a cultural group, understood but not openly discussed.

target population   The entire population to which the researcher wants to generalize the findings of a study.

telephone interview Interview to collect data conducted over the telephone instead of face-to-face.

terminus In prescriptive theory, the outcome of the procedure or intervention.

test A self-report measure in which the subject responds to individual items and achieves a total score intended to reflect the degree of the attribute held by the respondent.

testability Variables in a study that can be observed, measured, and analyzed.

test statistic A statistic used to test for the statistical significance of relationships, such as the chi-square or *t*-test.

testing effects A threat to the internal validity of a study in which change in the dependent variable is related to repeated testing; the effects of a pretest to responses on the post-test.

test–retest reliability An estimate of reliability of an instrument determined by comparing the results of testing at two points in time with the same individuals.

theme In qualitative research, a term used to describe the meaning of a recurring unit or category of data that is central to the presentation of the findings.

theoretical framework In research, the theory that generates research questions and hypotheses for testing and establishes a framework for the integration of research findings. Also called a theoretical model.

theoretical hypothesis See research hypothesis.

theoretical literature See conceptual literature.

theoretical model See theoretical framework.

theoretical notes Memos recorded by the researcher summarizing inductive or deductive thoughts about phenomena being observed in field studies.

theoretical propositions Theoretical statements that propose linkages between concepts to form theories.

theoretical sampling In qualitative research, sampling to improve representation of themes as the study evolves. Sampling is based on emerging findings and discovery of concepts with evidence of theoretical relevance to the evolving theory in grounded theory.

theoretical sensitivity The personal quality in a qualitative researcher that portrays an awareness of the subtleties of meaning embedded in the data.

theoretical simplicity Property in which a theory has the minimum number of interrelated components and is parsimonious.

theoretical term A complex abstract concept, with a meaning that is dependent on use in the theory.

theory A set of interrelated concepts and propositions that present a perspective on a phenomenon to describe, explain, or make predictions relative to the phenomenon.

theory-generating research Research designed to determine and describe phenomena and interrelationships among phenomena observed in the world.

theory-testing research Research that tests the accuracy of relationships described in a theory.

thick description In qualitative research, a thorough narrative description of the research context.

time sampling In observational studies, designation of the time points during which observations will occur.

time series analysis Method of analysis in which multiple observations of phenomena are made over time to determine and predict temporal patterns of variance.

time series design   A quasi-experimental longitudinal research design that includes multiple repeated observations at specific points in time and administration of an experimental treatment between two of the observations.

time-triggered strategies   Observational method in which observations are recorded at predetermined points of time.

topic guide   The researcher's list of questions or areas to discuss in a focus group or semistructured interview situation.

total variance   The true values and measurement errors that make up a score.

transferability   In qualitative research, a term to designate the probability that the research findings are meaningful or useful in other similar situations. Also called fittingness.

treatment   See experimental treatment.

treatment group   See experimental group.

treatment variable   See independent variable.

trend   An evaluation based on the increasing or decreasing slope or change of the data.

trend study   A longitudinal study that examines the slope of data collected over time from different samples in the population.

triangulation   The research approach of using multiple methods to collect data and information from subjects to understand and measure better the phenomenon of interest; combining both qualitative and quantitative methods in a study.

triangulation of data generation techniques   The use of three different methods to collect data in a study to generate a more complete data set.

triple-blind study A study in which the person interpreting results, the person providing the intervention, and the subject are unaware of the group assignment of participants.

true experimental design An experimental design in which the researcher manipulates an experimental variable, includes random assignment into groups, and includes a control group for comparison.

true variance The hypothetical true score or value determined under ideal conditions with no random error or measurement error.

trustworthiness In qualitative research, the establishment of the validity and reliability of the information to represent accurately the perceptions of the participants.

t-test A parametric statistical test for determining the difference between the means of two groups.

Tukey's test A post hoc statistical test used after a significant ANOVA to test differences in all possible pairs of means.

two-tailed hypothesis See nondirectional hypothesis.

two-tailed test A test of statistical significance in which both tails of the sampling distribution are examined in determining significance. The test is used when the direction of the relationship is unknown.

type I error The rejection of a null hypothesis that is actually true; a decision that a relationship exists between variables when it does not.

type II error The acceptance of a null hypothesis that is actually false; a decision that a relationship between variables does not exist when it does.

unimodal distribution A distribution with only one peak; one value occurs more frequently than any other.

unit of analysis The primary focus of a study, which can be an individual, group, family, community, organization, agency, or other social entity.

univariate Designs that include only one variable.

univariate descriptive study A study of one variable at a time to gather information on occurrence, frequency, and value of each variable without examination of the relationship between variables.

univariate statistics Descriptive statistics used to analyze one variable.

univariate study A research study in which only one variable is measured.

unstandardized interview An interview in which the interview process and procedures to collect data may differ between subjects.

unstructured interview A situation in which the interviewer does not follow a preset format and allows the participant to talk freely about the topic of interest.

unstructured observation The collection of information in which the researcher is guided by the research question to describe behaviors as they occur without a predetermined plan for collection and recording of the observations.

utility The property of being useful in a study or to the discipline.

utilization See research utilization.

utilization criteria The judgment of clinical relevance, scientific merit, and potential of an innovation to be implemented in the practice setting.

validation sample A sample that provides the initial data set for testing the reliability and validity of an instrument.

validity The degree to which an instrument measures what it is intended to measure.

validity coefficient An estimate of the validity of an instrument, ranging in value from .00 to 1.00.

validity of an estimate The degree to which an estimate of the population value differs from the true value of the population.

variability The degree of difference and distribution of values in a set of scores.

variable A characteristic or attribute of a phenomenon that differs within and among people or objects under study.

variance A summary of the variability of a distribution for data measured at the interval and ratio level of measurement. Variance is calculated by squaring each of the mathematical differences of each score from the mean and dividing the sum by the number of scores in the distribution. The standard deviation squared.

varimax method In factor analysis, a method to maximize the variance of the loadings within factors, across variables.

vignette A brief description of an event or situation to which subjects are asked to describe their opinion or response.

visual analog scale (VAS) An interval-level measure consisting of a straight line anchored at each end with the extreme limits of the attribute being measured. Participants select a point along the line that corresponds to the intensity of their experience.

voluntary sample A sample composed of people who request or volunteer to participate in a study.

volunteers Subjects who request or offer to participate in a study.

vulnerable subjects Groups of people who require special protection because of their inability to provide fully informed consent or because a circumstance or attribute places them more at risk than the general population. Examples of vulnerable subjects are children or people with some disabilities, mental illness or retardation, altered level of consciousness, or pregnancy.

Wald statistic A statistic used in logistic regression to evaluate the significance of individual predictors in the equation.

weighting A procedure to correct population values in a situation with a disproportionate sampling design.

Wilcoxon signed rank test A calculation of the difference between paired scores and a ranking of the difference.

Wilks' lambda A statistical test used in multivariate analyses to test the significance of group differences; measures the proportion of variance in the dependent variable not accounted for by any of the predictors.

within-group variation The variation in values within a data set obtained from the same group of participants.

within-subject analysis Analysis of the variation within data obtained from the same participant.

within-subjects design A research design in which an individual group of subjects is compared under different conditions or at different times.

X-axis The horizontal axis of a two-dimensional graph. Also called the abscissa.

Y-axis The vertical dimension of a two-dimensional graph. Also called the ordinate.

Yates' correction A correction to the chi-square statistic used when the frequency of less than 10 occurs for a cell in the contingency table.

zero-order correlation The correlation between two variables without controlling for the effects of other variables.

z score Scores expressed in terms of standard deviations from the mean of a set of values, with the scores from a normal distribution of values transformed to have a mean of 0 and a standard deviation of 1.0.

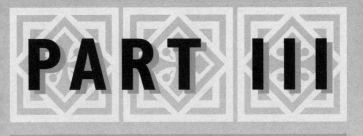

PART III

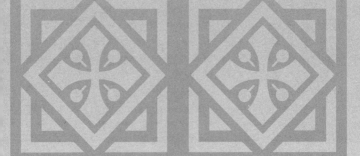

Compendium
of
Supplementary
Resources

Consent

••

Sample Consent Form

In signing this document, I am giving my consent to be interviewed by an employee of Humanalysis, Inc., a nonprofit research organization based in Saratoga Springs, New York. I understand that I will be part of a research study that will focus on the experiences and needs of mothers of young children in the United States. This study, supported by a grant from the U.S. Department of health and Human Services, will provide some guidance to people who are trying to help mothers and their children.

I understand that I will be interviewed in my home at a time convenient to me. I will be asked some questions about my experiences as a parent, my feelings about how to raise children, the health and characteristics of my oldest child, and my use of community services. I also understand that the interviewer will ask to have my oldest child present during at least some portion of the interview. The interview will take about $1\frac{1}{2}$ to 2 hours to complete. I also understand that the researcher may contact me for more information in the future.

I understand that I was selected to participate in this study because I was involved in a study of young mothers at the time of my oldest child's birth. At that time, I was recruited into the study, along with about 500 other young mothers, through a hospital or service agency.

This interview was granted freely. I have been informed that the interview is entirely voluntary, and that even after the interview begins I can refuse to answer any specific questions or decide to terminate the interview at any point. I have been told that my answers to questions will not be given to anyone else and no reports of this study will ever identify me in any way. I have also been informed that my participation or nonparticipation or my refusal to answer questions will have no effect on services that I or any member of my family may receive from health or social services providers.

This study will help develop a better understanding of the experiences of young mothers and the services that can be most helpful to them and their children. However, I will receive no direct benefit as a result of participation. As a means of compensating for any fatigue, inconvenience or monetary costs associated with participating in the study, I have received $25 for granting this interview.

I understand that the results of this research will be given to me if I ask for them and that Dr. Denise Polit is the person to contact if I have any questions about the study or about my rights as a study participant. Dr. Polit can be reached through a collect call at (518) 587-3994.

_____   _____
Date   Respondent's Signature

                                   _____
                                   Interviewer's Signature

Literature Review

A Quick Guide to Selected Abstracts and Indexes for Nursing and Related Subjects

Title	Type of Index		Frequency	Date Coverage	Subject Coverage			Types of Material Covered										Can Be Searched by Computer	
	Index	Abstract			Medicine	Nursing	Hospital	Other	Books	Studies	Technical report	Periodical	ANA/NLN Publ.	Gov't Publ.	Pamphlet	Dissertation	Book review	Data Base Name	Date
BOOKS																			
Card catalog of the library	●																		
National Library of Medicine current catalog @	●		Qa	1880	●	●	●		●	●	●		X	X	X	X		CATLINE	1801–
Catalog to the Sophia F. Palmer Memorial Library, AJN, Co.	●		2 vol.	1922–1973		●			●				●						
Medical Books in Print	●		A	1986	●	●	●	H	●									Books in Print	Current

(continued)

135

A Quick Guide to Selected Abstracts and Indexes for Nursing and Related Subjects (Continued)

Title	Abstract	Index	Frequency	Date Coverage	Medicine	Nursing	Hospital	Other	Books	Studies	Technical report	Periodical	ANA/NLN Publ.	Gov't Publ.	Pamphlet	Dissertation	Book review	Data Base Name	Date
PERIODICALS*																			
Annual or cumulative indexes to individual periodical titles (e.g., AJN, Public Health Nursing)		●			●	●						●	X	X	X		X		
International Nursing Index		●	Qa	1966		●			○			●	○	○	○	○		MEDLINE	1966–
CINAHL (Cumulative Index to Nursing and Allied Health Literature) @		●	B-Ma	1956		●			○			●	+	○	○			CINAHL	1983–

136

PERIODICALS

Source		Format	Dates	MEDLINE 1966–	HEALTH 1975–	BIOETHICS 1973–	HISTLINE 1970–	NTIS 1964–	MEDOC 1976–1979	Monthly catalog 1976–	Notes
Nursing Studies index (V. Henderson)	●	4 vol.	1900–1959	+							
Index Medicus/ Cumulated Index Medicus @	●	Ma	1927–	● +	+			+			
Hospital Literature Index/ Cumulative Index of Hospital Literature	●	Qa	1945	+	○	+	+	+ ●	●		H
History of Nursing Index to Adelaide Nutting, Teachers' College, Columbia U. collection	●			+ ×		+ ●	●				
Bibliography of Bioethics		1 vol. A	1973, 75–	+	+	● ●					M, e
Bibliography of the History of Medicine		Aa	1965–	+	+	+ +	●				

GOVERNMENT

Source		Format	Dates	MEDLINE 1966–	HEALTH 1975–	BIOETHICS 1973–	HISTLINE 1970–	NTIS 1964–	MEDOC 1976–1979	Monthly catalog 1976–	Notes
NTIS—SRIM Index to Health Planning	● ●	Qa	1978–					+			H
MEDOC		Qa	1968–					+	●		H
Monthly Catalog, U.S. Government Publications	●	Msa	1895–							●	M

(continued)

A Quick Guide to Selected Abstracts and Indexes for Nursing and Related Subjects (Continued)

Title	Index	Abstract	Frequency	Date Coverage	Medicine	Nursing	Hospital	Other	Books	Studies	Technical report	Periodical	ANA/NLN Publ.	Gov't Publ.	Pamphlet	Dissertation	Book review	Data Base Name	Date
ABSTRACTS																			
Annual Review of Nursing Research		●	A	1983–		●			+	+		+	X	X			+		
Nursing Abstracts		●	B-Ma	1979–		●						●							
Abstracts of Reports in Studies in Nursing (in each issue of *Nursing Research*)		●	B-M	1960–1978		●			+	●		+	+						
Abstracts of Studies in Public Health Nursing (in *Nursing Research*, 8, 1957)		●		1924–1957		●			+	●		+	+						

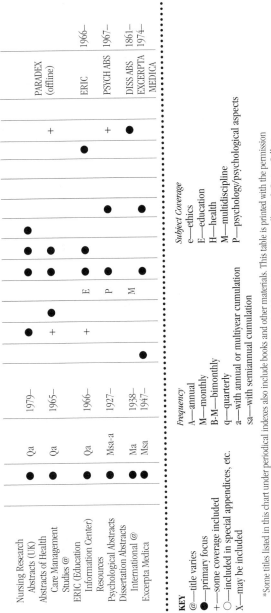

	Frequency		1979– / 1965– / 1966– / 1927– / 1938– / 1947–	Subject Coverage		PARADEX (offline)
Nursing Research Abstracts (UK)	Qa	●	1979–	●		
Abstracts of Health Care Management Studies @	Qa	●	1965–	+	● ●	
ERIC (Education Information Center) Resources	Qa	●	1966–	+	E	● ● ● ERIC 1966–
Psychological Abstracts	Msa-a	●	1927–	P	● ● ● +	PSYCH ABS 1967–
Dissertation Abstracts International @	Ma	● ●	1938–	M		DISS ABS 1861–
Excerpta Medica	Msa	●	1947–	●	● ● ● ●	EXCERPTA MEDICA 1974–

KEY

@—title varies
●—primary focus
+—some coverage included
○—included in special appendices, etc.
X—may be included

Frequency
A—annual
M—monthly
B-M—bimonthly
q—quarterly
a—with annual or multiyear cumulation
sa—with semiannual cumulation

Subject Coverage
e—ethics
E—education
H—health
M—multidiscipline
P—psychology/psychological aspects

*Some titles listed in this chart under periodical indexes also include books and other materials. This table is printed with the permission of its author, M. L. Pekarski, previously Coordinator, Special Projects, O'Neill Library (which contains a nursing collection), Boston College, Chestnut Hill, MA 02167.

Qualitative/Quantitative Perspectives

Major Assumptions of the Positivist and Naturalistic Paradigms

Philosophical Question	Positivist Paradigm Assumptions	Naturalistic Paradigm Assumptions
Ontologic (What is the nature of reality?)	Reality exists; there is a real world driven by real natural causes.	Reality is multiple and subjective, mentally constructed by individuals.
Epistemologic (How is the inquirer related to those being researched?)	Inquirer is independent from those being researched; the findings are not influenced by the researcher.	The inquirer interacts with those being researched; findings are the creation of the interactive process.
Axiologic (What is the role of values in the inquiry?)	Values and biases are to be held in check; objectivity is sought.	Subjectivity and values are inevitable and desirable.
Methodologic (How is knowledge obtained?)	Deductive processes Emphasis on discrete, specific concepts	Inductive processes Emphasis on entirety of some phenomenon, holistic
	Verification of researcher's hunches	Emerging interpretations grounded in participants' experiences
	Fixed design Tight controls over context	Flexible design Context-bound
	Emphasis on measured quantitative information; statistical analysis	Emphasis on narrative information; qualitative analysis
	Seeks generalizations	Seeks patterns

Research Purposes
and Research Questions

Purpose	Types of Questions: Quantitative Research	Types of Questions: Qualitative Research
Identification		What is this phenomenon? What is its name?
Description	How prevalent is the phenomenon? How often does the phenomenon occur? What are the characteristics of the phenomenon?	What are the dimensions of the phenomenon? What variations exist? What is important about the phenomenon?
Exploration	What factors are related to the phenomenon? What are the antecedents of the phenomenon?	What is the full nature of the phenomenon? What is really going on here? What is the process by which the phenomenon evolves or is experienced?
Explanation	What are the measurable associations between phenomena? What factors caused the phenomenon? Does the theory explain the phenomenon?	How does the phenomenon work? Why does the phenomenon exist? What is the meaning of the phenomenon? How did the phenomenon occur?
Prediction and control	What will happen if we alter a phenomenon or introduce an intervention? If phenomenon X occurs, will phenomenon Y follow? How can we make the phenomenon happen, or alter its nature or prevalence? Can the occurrence of the phenomenon be controlled?	

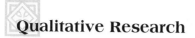

Qualitative Research

Critiquing Guidelines
for Qualitative Research

STATEMENT OF THE PHENOMENON OF INTEREST

1. Is the phenomenon of interest clearly identified?
2. Has the researcher identified why the phenomenon requires a qualitative format?
3. Are the philosophical underpinnings of the research described?

PURPOSE

1. Is the purpose of conducting the research made explicit?
2. Does the researcher describe the projected significance of the work to nursing?

METHOD

1. Is the method used to collect data compatible with the purpose of the research?
2. Is the method adequate to address the phenomenon of interest?

SAMPLING

1. Does the researcher describe the selection of participants? Is purposive sampling used?
2. Are the informants who were chosen appropriate to inform the research?

DATA COLLECTION

1. Is data collection focused on human experience?
2. Does the researcher describe data collection strategies? [i.e., interview, observation, field notes]
3. Is protection of human subjects addressed?
4. Is saturation of the data described?
5. Are the procedures for collecting data made explicit?

DATA ANALYSIS

1. Does the researcher describe the strategies used to analyze the data?
2. Has the researcher remained true to the data?
3. Does the reader understand the procedures used to analyze the data?
4. Does the researcher address the credibility, auditability, and fittingness of the data?

   Credibility

   a. Do the participants recognize the experience as their own?

Auditability
a. Can the reader follow the thinking of the researcher?
b. Does the researcher document the research process?

Fittingness
a. Can the findings be applicable outside of the study situation?
b. Are the results meaningful to individuals not involved in the research?

5. Is the strategy used for analysis compatible with the purpose of the study?

Findings
1. Are the findings presented within a context?
2. Is the reader able to apprehend the essence of the experience from the report of the findings?
3. Are the researcher's conceptualizations true to the data?
4. Does the researcher place the report in the context of what is already known about the phenomenon?

Conclusions, Implications, and Recommendations
1. Do the conclusions, implications and recommendations give the reader a context in which to use the findings?
2. Do the conclusions reflect the findings of the study?
3. Are recommendations for future study offered?
4. Is the significance of the study to nursing made explicit?

. . . .

Source: Streubert, H. (1994). Evaluating the qualitative research report. In G. Lo-Biondo-Wood & J. Haber, (Eds.). *Nursing research: Methods, critical appraisal, and utilization* (3rd. ed.). (pp. 481–499). St. Louis: Mosby.

Historical Research Questions to Be Addressed

....

GENERATION OF DATA

Title

1. How does it concisely reflect the purpose of the study?
2. How does it clearly tell the reader what the study is about?
3. How does it delineate the time frame for the study?

Statement of the Subject

1. Is the subject easily researched?
2. What themes and theses are studied?
3. What are the research questions?
4. Are there primary sources available to study the subject?
5. Has it been studied before?
6. What makes this study different or similar than others?
7. What is the significance to nursing?
8. What is the rationale for the time frame for the study?

Literature Review

1. What are the main works written on the subject?
2. What time period does the literature review cover?
3. What are some of the problems that may arise when studying this subject?
4. Can primary sources be identified?
5. Was the subject narrowed during the literature review?
6. What research questions were raised during the literature review?

TREATMENT OF DATA

Primary Sources

1. How were primary sources used?
2. Were they genuine and authentic?
3. How was external validity determined?
4. How was internal validity determined?
5. Were there inconsistencies between the external validity and internal validity?
6. Does the content accurately reflect the period of concern?
7. Do the facts conflict with historical dates, meanings of words, and social mores?
8. When did the primary author write the account?
9. Did a trained historian or an observer author the source?
10. Were facts suppressed, and if so, why?
11. Is there corroborating evidence?
12. Identify any disagreements between sources.

Secondary Sources
1. What were the secondary sources used?
2. How were secondary sources used?
3. Do they corroborate the primary source?
4. Can you identify any disagreements between sources?

DATA ANALYSIS
Organization
1. What conceptual frameworks were used in the study?
2. How would the study be classified: intellectual, feminist, social, political, biographical?
3. Were the research questions answered?
4. Was the purpose of the study accomplished?
5. If conflict exists within the findings, was there supporting evidence to justify either side of the argument?

Bias
1. Was the researcher's bias identified?
2. Was analysis influenced by a present-mindedness?
3. What were the ideological biases?
4. How did bias affect the analysis of the data?

Ethical Issue
1. Was there any infringement on historical reputation?
2. Was there a conflict between the right to privacy versus the right to know?
3. Did the research show that decisions, events, and activities of an individual or organization affected the public welfare or embraced qualities of major human interest?

INTERPRETING THE FINDINGS
Narrative
1. Does the story describe what happened, including how and why it happened?
2. Were relations between events, ideas, people, organizations, and institutions explained, interpreted, and placed within a contextual framework?
3. How were direct quotations used (too limited or too long)?
4. Was the narrative clear, concise, and interesting to read?
5. Was the significance to nursing explicit?

Steps for Conducting Ethnographic Research

Doing participant observation

Making an ethnographic record

Making descriptive observations

Making a domain analysis

Making focused observation

Making a taxonomic analysis

Making selected observations

Making a componential analysis

Discovering cultural themes

Taking a cultural inventory

Writing an ethnography

Guidelines for Critiquing Research Using Grounded Theory Method

STATEMENT OF THE PHENOMENON OF INTEREST

1. Is the phenomenon of interest clearly identified?
2. Has the researcher identified why the phenomenon requires a qualitative format?

PURPOSE

1. Is the purpose for conducting the research made explicit?
2. Does the researcher describe the projected significance of the work to nursing?

METHOD

1. Is the method used to collect data compatible with the purpose of the research?

SAMPLING

1. Does the researcher describe the selection of participants?
2. What major categories emerged?
3. What were some of the events, incidents, and/or actions that pointed to some of these major categories?
4. What were the categories that led to theoretical sampling?
5. After the theoretical sampling was done, how representative did the categories prove to be?

DATE GENERATION

1. Does the researcher describe data collection strategies?
2. How did theoretical formulations guide data collection?

DATA ANALYSIS

1. Does the researcher describe the strategies used to analyze the data?
2. Does the researcher address the credibility, auditability, and fittingness of the data?
3. Does the researcher clearly describe how and why the core category was selected?

EMPIRICAL GROUNDING OF THE STUDY—FINDINGS

1. Are concepts grounded in the data?
2. Are the concepts systematically related?
3. Are conceptual linkages described and are the categories well developed? Do they have conceptual density?
4. Are the theoretical findings significant and to what extent?

(continued)

Guidelines for Critiquing Research
Using Grounded Theory Method (Continued)
• •

   5. Was data collection comprehensive and analytical interpretations conceptual and broad?

   6. Is there sufficient variation to allow for applicability in a variety of contexts related to the phenomenon investigated?

CONCLUSIONS, IMPLICATIONS, AND RECOMMENDATIONS

   1. Do the conclusions, implications, and recommendations give the reader a context in which to use the findings?

   2. Do the conclusions reflect the findings of the study?

   3. Are recommendations for future study offered?

   4. Is the significance of the study to nursing made explicit?
• •

Adapted from: Streubert, H. (1994). Evaluating the qualitative research report. In G. W. LoBiondo & J. Haber (Eds.), *Nursing research: Methods, critical appraisal, and utilization,* 3rd ed. (pp. 481–499). St. Louis: Mosby; and Strauss, A., & Corbin, J. (1990). *Basics of qualitative research: Grounded theory procedures and techniques.* Newbury Park, CA: Sage Publications.

Quantitative Research

Dimensions of Quantitative Research Designs

Dimension	Design	Major Features
Control over independent variable	• Experimental	Manipulation of independent variable, control group, randomization
	• Quasi-experimental	Manipulation of independent variable but no randomization or no control group
	• Nonexperimental	No manipulation of independent variable
Type of group comparisons	• Between-subjects	Participants in groups being compared are different people
	• Within-subjects	Participants in groups being compared are the same people
Number of data collection points	• Cross-sectional	Data collected at one point in time
	• Longitudinal	Data collected at multiple points in time over extended period
Occurrence of independent and dependent variable	• Retrospective	Study begins with dependent variable and looks backward for cause or influence
	• Prospective	Study begins with independent variable and looks forward for the effect
Setting	• Naturalistic	Data collected in a real-world setting
	• Laboratory	Data collected in artificial, contrived setting

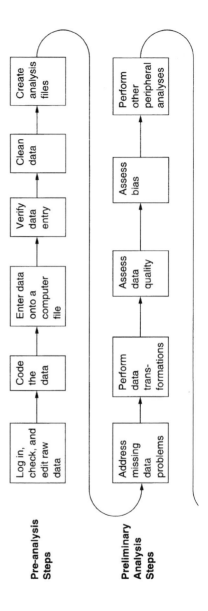

Pre-analysis Steps

Log in, check, and edit raw data → Code the data → Enter data onto a computer file → Verify data entry → Clean data → Create analysis files

Preliminary Analysis Steps

Address missing data problems → Perform data transformations → Assess data quality → Assess bias → Perform other peripheral analyses

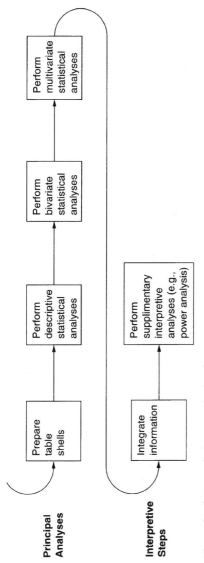

Principal Analyses

Prepare table shells

Perform descriptive statistical analyses

Perform bivariate statistical analyses

Perform multivariate statistical analyses

Interpretive Steps

Integrate information

Perform supplimentary interpretive analyses (e.g., power analysis)

Flow of tasks in analyzing quantitative data

Instruments

Fictitious Example of a Cover Letter for a Mailed Questionnaire

Dear _____:

We are conducting a study to examine how women who are approaching retirement age (age 55 to 65) feel about various issues relating to health and health care. This study, which is sponsored by the State Department of Health, will enable health-care providers to better meet the needs of women in your age group. Would you please assist us in this study by completing the enclosed questionnaire? Your opinions and experiences are very important to us and are needed to give an accurate picture of the health-related needs of women in the greater Middletown area.

Your name was selected at random from a list of residents in your community. The questionnaire is completely anonymous, so you are not asked to put your name on it or to identify yourself in any way. We therefore hope that you will feel comfortable about giving your honest opinions. If you prefer not to answer any particular question, please feel perfectly free to leave it blank. Please do answer the questions if you can, though, and if you have any comments or concerns about any question, just write your comments in the margin.

A postage-paid return envelope has been provided for your convenience. We hope that you will take a few minutes to complete and return the questionnaire to us—it should take only about 15 minutes of your time. To analyze the information in a timely fashion, we ask that you return the questionnaire to us by May 12.

Thank you very much for your cooperation and assistance in this endeavor. If you would like a copy of the summary of the results of this study, please check the box at the bottom of page 10.

Examples of Question Types

• •

OPEN-ENDED

1. What led to your decision to stop using oral contraceptives?
2. What did you do when you discovered you had AIDS?

CLOSED-ENDED

1. Dichotomous Question
   Have you ever been hospitalized?
   ( ) 1. Yes
   ( ) 2. No
2. Multiple-Choice Question
   How important is it to you to avoid a pregnancy at this time?
   ( ) 1. Extremely important
   ( ) 2. Very important
   ( ) 3. Somewhat important
   ( ) 4. Not at all important
3. "Cafeteria" Question
   People have different opinions about the use of estrogen-replacement
   therapy for women in menopause. Which of the following statements
   best represents your point of view?
   ( ) 1. Estrogen replacement is dangerous and should be totally
           banned.
   ( ) 2. Estrogen replacement may have some undesirable side ef-
           fects that suggest the need for caution in its use.
   ( ) 3. I am undecided about my views on estrogen-replacement
           therapy.
   ( ) 4. Estrogen replacement has many beneficial effects that merit
           its promotion.
   ( ) 5. Estrogen replacement is a wonder cure that should be ad-
           ministered routinely to menopausal women.
4. Rank-Order Question
   People value different things about life. Below is a list of principles or
   ideals that are often cited when people are asked to name things they
   value most. Please indicate the order of importance of these values to
   you by placing a *1* beside the most important, *2* beside the next most
   important, and so forth.
   ( ) Achievement and success
   ( ) Family relationships
   ( ) Friendships and social interaction
   ( ) Health
   ( ) Money
   ( ) Religion

(continued)

Examples of Question Types (Continued)

5. Forced-Choice Question

   Which statement most closely represents your point of view?

   ( ) 1. What happens to me is my own doing.

   ( ) 2. Sometimes, I feel I don't have enough control over my life.

6. Rating Question

   On a scale from 0 to 10, where 0 means extremely dissatisfied and 10 means extremely satisfied, how satisfied are you with the nursing care you received during your hospitalization?

   Extremely dissatisfied   Extremely satisfied

   0   1   2   3   4   5   6   7   8   9   10

Examples of Concepts Frequently Measured With Composite Scales

●●

Concept	Research Example Reference	Instrument Used
Anxiety	Erler & Rudman, 1993	State-Trait Anxiety Inventory (STAI)
	Littlefield, Chang, & Adams, 1990	Multiple Affect Adjective Adjective Checklist
Body image	Nicholas & Leuner, 1992	Body Cathexis Scale (BCS)
	Mock, 1993	Body Image Scale
Coping	Hahn, Brooks, & Hartsough, 1993	Lazarus Ways of Coping Scale
	Herth, 1990	Jalowiec Coping Scale
Depression	Fogel, 1993	Center for Epidemiological Studies Depression Scale (CES-D)
	Buchanan, Cowan, Burr , Waldron, & Kogan, 1993	Beck Depression Inventory (BDI)
Family functioning	Stuifbergen, 1990	Family Environment Scale (FES)
	Woods, Haberman, & Packard, 1993	Family Adaptability & Cohesion Evaluation Scales (FACES)
Hope	Farran, Salloway, & Clark, 1990	Stoner Hope Scale
	Christman, 1990	Beck Hopelessness Scale
Life satisfaction	Topp & Stevenson, 1994	Life Satisfaction Scale (LSS)
	Foster, 1992	Life Satisfaction Index (LSI)
Mood states	Crumlish, 1994	Profile of Mood States (POMS)
	King, Porter, Norsen, & Reis, 1992	Bipolar Profile of Mood States (POMS-BI)
Pain	Neill, 1993	McGill Pain Questionnaire
Psychosomatic symptoms	Cossette & Levesque, 1993	Symptom Checklist-90 (SCL-90)

(continued)

Examples of Concepts Frequently
Measured With Composite Scales (Continued)

Concept	Research Example Reference	Instrument Used
Self-care agency	Jirovec & Kasno, 1993 Behm & Frank, 1992	Appraisal of Self Care Agency Exercise of Self-Care Agency (ESCA)
Self-esteem	Weaver & Narsavage, 1992 Walsh, 1993	Rosenberg Self-Esteem Scale Coopersmith Self-Esteem Inventory
Social support	White, Richter, & Fry, 1992 Dodd, Dibble, & Thomas, 1993	Personal Resource Question- naire (PRQ85) Norbeck Social Support Questionnaire
Stress	Gardner, 1991 Gennaro, Brooten, Roncoli, & Kumar, 1993	Hospital Stress Rating Scale Life Experiences Survey

NURSE PRACTITIONERS

	7*	6	5	4	3	2	1	
competent								incompetent
worthless	1	2	3	4	5	6	7	valuable
important								unimportant
pleasant								unpleasant
bad								good
cold								warm
responsible								irresponsible
successful								unsuccessful

*The score values would not be printed on the form administered to actual subjects. The numbers are presented here solely for the purpose of illustrating how semantic differentials are scored.

Example of a semantic differential

157

Example of a Likert Scale to Measure Attitudes Toward the Mentally Ill

Direction of Scoring*	Item	Responses†					Score	
		SA	A	?	D	SD	Person 1 (✓)	Person 2 (X)
+	1. People who have had a mental illness can become normal, productive citizens after treatment.		✓			X	4	1
−	2. People who have been patients in mental hospitals should not be allowed to have children.			X		✓	5	3
−	3. The best way to handle patients in mental hospitals is to restrict their activity as much as possible.		X		✓		4	2
+	4. Many patients in mental hospitals develop normal, healthy relationships with staff members and other patients.			✓	X		3	2
+	5. There should be an expanded effort to get the mentally ill out of institutional settings and back into their communities.	✓				X	5	1
−	6. Because the mentally ill cannot be trusted, they should be kept under constant guard.		X			✓	5	2
TOTAL SCORE							26	11

*Researchers would not indicate the direction of scoring on a Likert scale administered to subjects. The scoring direction is indicated in this table for illustrative purposes only.

†SA, strongly agree; A, agree; ?, uncertain; D, disagree; SD, strongly disagree.

Here are some characteristics of birth-control devices that are of varying importance to different people. How important a consideration has each of these been for you in choosing a birth-control method?

	Of Very Great Importance	Of Great Importance	Of Some Importance	Of No Importance
1. Comfort				
2. Cost				
3. Ease of use				
4. Effectiveness				
5. Noninterference with spontaneity				
6. Safety to you				
7. Safety to partner				

Example of a checklist

Statistical Information

Summary of Statistical Tests

Name of Procedure	Test Statistic	Degrees of Freedom	Purpose	Parametric (P) or Non-Parametric (NP)	Levels of Measurement	
					Variable 1 (Independent)	Variable 2 (Dependent)
t-Test for independent samples	t	$n_{Group A} + n_{Group B} - 2$	To test the difference between the means of two independent groups	P	Nominal	Interval or ratio
t-Test for dependent (paired) samples	t	$n - 1$	To test the difference between the means of two related groups or sets of scores	P	Nominal	Interval or ratio
Median Test	χ^2	(Rows −1) × (Columns − 1)	To test the difference between the medians of two independent groups	NP	Nominal	Ordinal
Mann-Whitney U Test	U (Z)	$n - 1$	To test the difference in the ranks of scores of two independent groups	NP	Nominal	Ordinal

Wilcoxon Signed-Rank Test	Z	$n - 2$	NP	To test the difference in the ranks of scores of two related groups or sets of scores	Nominal	Ordinal
ANOVA	F	Between: n of groups $- 1$ Within: n of subjects $- n$ of groups	P	To test the difference among the means of three or more independent groups, or of more than one independent variable	Nominal	Interval or ratio
Kruskal-Wallis Test	H (χ^2)	n of groups $- 1$	NP	To test the difference in the ranks of scores of three or more independent groups	Nominal	Ordinal
Friedman Test	χ^2	n of groups $- 1$	NP	To test the difference in the ranks of scores for three or more related sets of scores	Nominal	Ordinal
Chi-Square Test	χ^2	$(\text{Rows} - 1) \times (\text{Columns} - 1)$	NP	To test the difference in proportion in two or more groups	Nominal	Nominal
McNemar's Test	χ^2	1	NP	To test the differences in proportions for paired samples (2×2)	Nominal	Nominal
Fisher's Exact Test	†	†	NP	To test the difference in proportions in a 2×2 contingency table when $N < 30$	Nominal	Nominal

(continued)

161

Summary of Statistical Tests (Continued)

Name of Procedure	Test Statistic	Degrees of Freedom	Parametric (P) or Non-Parametric (NP)	Purpose	Variable 1 (Independent)	Variable 2 (Dependent)
					Levels of Measurement	
Pearson Product-moment correlation	r	$n-2$	P	To test that a correlation is different from zero (i.e., that a relationship exists)	Interval or ratio	Interval or ratio
Spearman's rho	ρ	$n-2$	NP	To test that a correlation is different from zero (i.e., that a relationship exists)	Ordinal	Ordinal
Kendall's tau	τ	$n-2$	NP	To test that a correlation is different from zero (i.e., that a relationship exists)	Ordinal	Ordinal
Phi coefficient	ϕ	1*	NP	To examine the magnitude of a relationship between two dichotomous variables (2×2)	Nominal	Nominal
Cramer's V	V	$(R-1) \times (C-1)$*	NP	To examine the magnitude of a relationship between variables in a contingency table (not restricted to 2×2)	Nominal	Nominal

*The test that $\phi \neq 0$ (or $V \neq 0$) is provided by the χ^2 test.
†Fisher's Exact Test computes exact probabilities directly.

Guide to Widely Used Multivariate Statistical Analyses

		Measurement Level*			Number of:		
Name	Purpose	IV	DV	Cov	IVs	DVs	Covs
Multiple correlation/ regression	To test the relationship between 2+ IVs and 1 DV; to predict a DV from 2+ IVs	N,I,R	I,R		2+	1	
Analysis of covariance (ANCOVA)	To test the difference between the means of 2+ groups, while controlling for 1+ covariate	N	I,R	N,I,R	1+	1	1+
Multivariate analysis of variance (MANOVA)	To test the difference between the means of 2+ groups for 2+ DVs simultaneously	N	I,R		1+	2+	
Multivariate analysis of covariance (MANCOVA)	To test the difference between the means of 2+ groups for 2+ DVs simultaneously, while controlling for 1+ covariate	N	I,R	N,I,R	1+	2+	1+

(continued)

Guide to Widely Used Multivariate Statistical Analyses (Continued)

| Name | Purpose | Measurement Level* | | | Number of: | | |
		IV	DV	Cov	IVs	DVs	Covs
Canonical analysis	To test the relationship between two sets of variables (variables on the right, variables on the left)	N,I,R	N,I,R		2+	2+	
Factor analysis	To determine the dimensionality/structure of a set of variables						
Discriminant analysis	To test the relationship between 2+ IVs and 1 DV; to predict group membership; to classify cases into groups	N,I,R	N		2+	1	
Logistic regression	To test the relationship between 2+ IVs and 1 DV; to predict the probability of an event; to estimate relative risk (odds ratios)	N,I,R	N		2+	1	

*Measurement level of the independent variable (IV), dependent variable (DV), and covariates (COV): N = nominal, I = interval, R = ratio.

Computerized Qualitative Data Management Programs

••

Computer Program	Source
MS-DOS Programs	
Atlas-Ti	Qualitative Research Management 73425 Hilltop Road Desert Hot Springs, CA 92241 (619) 320–7026
Ethnograph (Version 3.0)	Qualis Research Associates P.O. Box 2070 Amherst, MA 01004 (415) 256–8835 $150.00
Hyper Research for Windows	Qualitative Research Management 73425 Hilltop Road Desert Hot Springs, CA 92241 (619) 320–7026 $275.00
Martin (Version 2.0)	Martin School of Nursing University of Wisconsin-Madison 600 Highland Avenue Madison, WI 53792 (608) 263–5336 $250.00
Textbase Alpha	Qualitative Research Management 73425 Hilltop road Desert Hot Springs, CA 92241 (619) 320–7026 $150.00
Macintosh Programs	
HyperQual 2	Qualitative Research Management 73425 Hilltop Road Desert Hot Springs, CA 92241 (619) 320–7026 $180.00

(continued)

Computerized Qualitative Data
Management Programs (Continued)

••

Computer Program	Source
Macintosh Programs	
Hyper Soft	Qualitative Research Management 73425 Hilltop Road Desert Hot Springs, CA 92241 (619) 320–7026 $175.00
Nudist (Version 3.0)	Learning Profiles, Inc. 2329 W. Main Street, #330 Littleton, CO 80120–1951 (800) 279–2070 $275.00

••

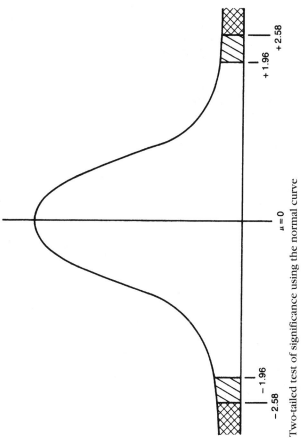

Two-tailed test of significance using the normal curve

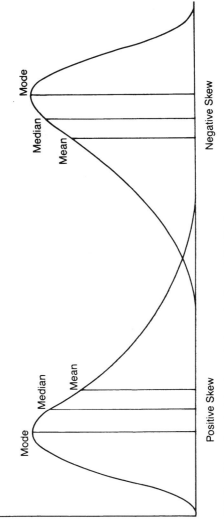

Relationships of central tendency indexes in skewed distributions

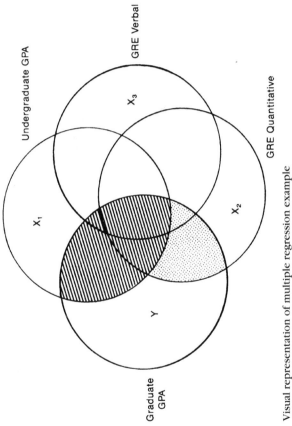

Visual representation of multiple regression example

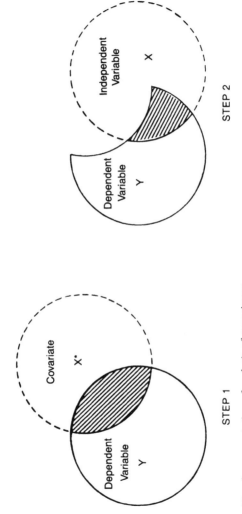

Visual representation of analysis of covariance

The actual situation is that the null hypothesis is:

	True	False
True (Null accepted)	Correct decision	Type II error
False (Null rejected)	Type I error	Correct decision

The researcher calculates a test statistic and decides that the null hypothesis is:

Outcomes of statistical decision making

Guidelines for the Preparation of Tables

- A table makes it possible to compare and comprehend patterns and relationships among data. Most quantitative studies benefit from the inclusion of one or more tables, but tables should be reserved for important substantive information that is too cumbersome to report in the text. Avoid very short tables, such as a table with two columns and two rows; it is more efficient to present such information in the text.
- Tables are effective only when the data are arranged in such a way that the patterns are obvious at a glance. Care needs to be taken in organizing the information in an intelligible way.
- If there is a choice between what to put on the horizontal and vertical dimensions of the table, keep in mind that it is easier for readers to compare numbers down a column than across a row.
- Every column of data should have a heading. Table headings should establish the logic of the table structure. The headings should be succinct but clear.
- Numerical values should be expressed in the number of decimal places justified by the precision of measurement. However, it is often preferable to report numbers in tables to a maximum of one decimal place (except correlation coefficients); rounded numbers are often easier to absorb and compare than more precise values. The number of decimal places should be the same across entries in the table.
- Probability values should be clearly indicated, as appropriate, either by indicating the actual p values or by using asterisks and a probability level note. When more than one probability level is indicated in the table, use one asterisk for the least stringent level, two for the next level, and so on (e.g., $*p < .05$, $**p < .01$). It is not necessary to use the same probability levels and number of asterisks from one table to the next.
- Every table should be comprehensible without reference to the text. All abbreviations (except commonly used ones such as N or SD) and special symbols should be explained in notes to the table.
- When applicable, the units of measurement for the numbers in the table should always be indicated e.g., pounds, dollars, beats per minute, milligrams, etc.).
- Each table should be referred to in the text (e.g., "As shown in Table 2, patients who . . ."). Thus, every table should be numbered.
- Every table should have a clear, but brief, explanatory title.

Critique Guidelines

Guidelines for the Conduct of a Written Research Critique

1. Be sure to comment on the study's strengths as well as its weaknesses. The critique should be a balanced consideration of the worth of the research. Each research report has at least *some* positive features—be sure to find them and note them.

2. Give specific examples of the study's weaknesses and strengths. Avoid vague generalities of praise and fault finding.

3. Try to justify your criticisms. Offer a rationale for how a different approach would have solved a problem that the researcher failed to address.

4. Be as objective as possible. Try to avoid being overly critical of a study because you are not particularly interested in the topic or because you have a bias against a certain research approach (e.g., qualitative vs. quantitative).

5. Without sacrificing objectivity, be sensitive in handling negative comments. Try to put yourself in the shoes of the researcher receiving the critical appraisal. Try not to be condescending or sarcastic.

6. Suggest alternatives that the researcher (or future researchers) might want to consider. Do not just identify the problems in the research study—offer some recommended solutions, making sure that the recommendations are practical ones.

7. Evaluate all aspects of the study—its substantive, methodological, interpretive, ethical, and presentational dimensions.

Guidelines for Critiquing Problem Statements and Hypotheses

1. Does the research report clearly present the research problem? Was the problem statement introduced promptly? Was it placed in a logical and easy-to-find location?
2. Does the problem have significance to the nursing profession, and does the researcher describe what that significance is?
3. Does the problem seem sensible and justifiable? Does it flow from prior scientific information, experience in the topic area, or a theory? In the context of current knowledge on the topic, is the problem the right one to address?
4. Has the researcher appropriately delimited the scope of the problem, or is the problem too big or complex for a single investigation?
5. Does the problem statement clearly identify the research variables and the nature of the population being studied? Are the research variables adequately defined? Is the problem statement clearly and concisely articulated?
6. Does the research report contain formally stated hypotheses? If not, is their absence justifiable? Are the hypotheses directly and logically tied to the research problems?
7. Do the hypotheses flow logically from the theoretical framework or from prior research? If not, is adequate justification offered for the researcher's predictions?
8. Can the hypotheses be tested in such a way that it is clear whether the hypotheses are supported?
9. Are the hypotheses properly worded? Does each hypothesis express a predicted relationship between two or more variables? Are they worded clearly and objectively and written as a stated prediction?
10. Are the hypotheses stated as research hypotheses rather than as null hypotheses? Are the hypotheses directional? If not, is there a rationale for the nondirectional hypotheses?

Guidelines for Critiquing Research Designs

1. Given the nature of the research question, what type of design is most appropriate? How much flexibility does the research question call for, and how much structure is needed?

2. Does the design involve an experimental intervention? Was the full nature of any intervention described in detail?

3. If there is an intervention, was a true experimental, quasi-experimental, or preexperimental design used? Should a more rigorous design have been used?

4. If the design is nonexperimental, what is the reason that the researcher decided not to manipulate the independent variable? Was this decision appropriate?

5. What types of comparisons are specified in the research design (e.g., before–after, the use of one or more comparison group)? Are these comparisons the most appropriate ones?

6. If the research design does not call for any comparisons, what difficulties, if any, does this pose for understanding what the results mean?

7. How many times were data collected or observations recorded? Is this number appropriate, given the research questions?

8. What procedures, if any, did the researcher use to control external (situational) factors? Were these procedures appropriate and adequate?

9. What procedures, if any, did the researcher use to control extraneous subject characteristics? Were these procedures appropriate and adequate?

10. To what extent did the design affect the internal validity of the study? What alternative explanations must be considered, given the design that was used?

11. To what extent did the design enhance the external validity of the study? Can the design be criticized for its artificiality, or praised for its realism?

12. Does the research design enable the researcher to draw causal inferences about the relationships among research variables?

13. What are the major limitations of the design used? Are these limitations acknowledged by the researcher?

Guidelines for Critiquing Quantitative Analyses

1. Do the research data lend themselves to quantitative analysis? Would a qualitative approach to data analysis have been more appropriate?

2. Does the report include any descriptive statistics? Do these statistics sufficiently describe the major characteristics of the researcher's data set?

3. Were indices of both central tendency and variability provided in the report? If not, how does the absence of this information affect the reader's understanding of the research variables?

4. Were the correct descriptive statistics used (e.g., was a median used when a mean would have been more appropriate?

5. Does the report include any inferential statistics? Was a statistical test performed for each of the hypotheses or research questions? If inferential statistics were not used, should they have been?

6. Was the selected statistical test appropriate, given the level of measurement of the variables?

7. Was a parametric test used? Does it appear that the assumptions for the use of parametric tests were met? If a nonparametric test was used, should a more powerful parametric procedure have been used instead?

8. Were any multivariate procedures used? If so, does it appear that the researcher chose the appropriate test? If multivariate procedures were not used, should they have been? Would the use of a multivariate procedure have improved the researcher's ability to draw conclusions about the relationship between the dependent and independent variables?

9. In general, does the research report provide a rationale for the researcher's decision to use certain statistical tests but not others? Does the report contain sufficient information for the reader to judge whether appropriate statistics were used?

10. Was there an appropriate amount of statistical information reported? Are the findings clearly and logically organized?

11. Were the results of any statistical tests significant? What do the tests tell the reader about the plausibility of the research hypotheses?

12. Were tables used judiciously to summarize large masses of statistical information? Are the tables clearly presented, with good titles and carefully labeled column headings? Is the information presented in the text consistent with the information presented in the tables? Is the information totally redundant?

13. Could the study have been strengthened by the inclusion of some qualitative data?

Guidelines for Critiquing Qualitative Analyses

••

1. Are the data best analyzed qualitatively, or would a quantitative approach have been more appropriate?

2. Is the research tradition within which the study was undertaken identified (e.g., ethnographic, phenomenological)? Do the methods of data collection and analysis appear to be congruent with this tradition?

3. What sources of data were used to yield the qualitative materials (e.g., unstructured interview, observation)? Are these sources sufficient to provide a broad array of information and to capture the full range of likely variation regarding the phenomenon under investigation?

4. Are the coding categories used to organize the data described? Are examples of data fitting each category presented? Does the report describe the rules used to place data into the categories? Do the categories seem to be logical and complete? Does there seem to be unnecessary overlap or redundancy in the categories?

5. Is the reasoning process through which the thematic analysis occurred clearly described? What were the major themes that emerged? If excerpts from the narrative materials are provided, do these themes appear to capture the meaning of the narratives (i.e., did the researcher adequately interpret and conceptualize the themes)?

6. Is the analysis parsimonious? That is, could two or more themes have been collapsed into some broader and perhaps more useful conceptualization of the issues?

7. What efforts did the researcher make to validate the findings? Were quasi-statistical procedures used? Did two or more researchers independently code and analyze the data? Did the researcher specifically mention a search for contrary occurrences? What evidence does the report provide that the researcher's analysis is accurate, objective, and replicable?

8. Was the grounded theory approach used? If so, does it appear to have been used appropriately? Did data collection continue until saturation occurred? Were data collection and analysis undertaken concurrently?

9. Were the data displayed in a manner that allows the reader to verify the researcher's theoretical conclusions? Was a conceptual map or framework displayed to communicate important processes?

10. Was the context of the phenomenon under investigation adequately described? Does the report give the reader a clear picture of the social world of those people under study?

(continued)

Guidelines for Critiquing
Qualitative Analyses (Continued)

11. Does the theoretical schema yield a meaningful picture of the phenomenon under study? Are the relationships among the concepts clearly expressed? Do these relationships seem logical, and do they accurately reflect the data? Is the resulting theory trivial and obvious?

12. Could the study have been strengthened by the inclusion of some quantitative data?

Guidelines for Critiquing the Interpretive Dimensions of a Research Report

INTERPRETATION OF THE FINDINGS

1. Are all the important results discussed? Are the interpretations consistent with the results?
2. Is each result interpreted in terms of the original hypothesis to which it relates and to the conceptual framework? Is each result interpreted in light of findings from similar research studies?
3. Are alternative explanations for the findings mentioned, and is the rationale for their rejection discussed?
4. Do the interpretations give due consideraton to the limitations of the research methods?
5. Are any unwarranted interpretations of causality made?
6. Is there evidence of bias in the interpretations?
7. Does the interpretation distinguish between practical and statistical significance?

IMPLICATIONS

8. Are implications of the study ignored, although a basis for them is apparent?
9. Are the implications of the study discussed in terms of the retention, modification, or rejection of a theory or conceptual framework?
10. Are the implications of the findings for nursing practice described?
11. Are the discussed implications appropriate, given the study's limitations?
12. Are generalizations made that are not warranted on the basis of the sample used?

RECOMMENDATIONS

13. Are recommendations made concerning how the study's methods could be impoved? Are recommendations for future research investigations made?
14. Are recommendations for specific nursing actions made on the basis of the implications?
15. Are the recommendations thorough, consistent with the findings, and consistent with related research results?

Guidelines for Critiquing the Ethical Aspects of a Study

1. Were the subjects unnecessarily subjected to any physical harm or psychological distress or discomfort?
2. Did the researchers take appropriate steps to remove or prevent harm?
3. Did the benefits that accrued from the research outweigh any potential risks or actual discomfort to the subjects?
4. Was information gathered from study participants by personnel with appropriate qualifications?
5. Were the subjects told about any real or potential risks that might result from participation in the study? Were the purposes and procedures of the study fully described in advance?
6. Was any type of coercion or undue influence used in recruiting subjects for the study? Were vulnerable subjects used?
7. Did all the subjects know they were subjects in a study? Did they have an opportunity to decline participation? Were subjects deceived in any way?
8. Was informed consent obtained from all subjects or their representatives? If not, was there a valid and justifiable reason for not doing so?
9. Were appropriate steps taken to safeguard the privacy of the research subjects?
10. Was the research study approved and monitored by an Institutional Review Board or other similar committee on ethics?

Index

181